Solo Training
The Martial Artist's Guide to Training Alone

Solo Training
The Martial Artist's Guide to Training Alone

by
Loren W. Christensen

YMAA Publication Center, Inc.
Wolfeboro, NH USA

YMAA Publication Center, Inc.
PO Box 480
Wolfeboro, NH 03894
800 669-8892 • www.ymaa.com • info@ymaa.com

Paperback ISBN: 9781594394881 (print) • ISBN: 9781594394898 (ebook)

20200407

Publisher's Cataloging in Publication

Christensen, Loren W.
    Solo training : the martial artist's guide to training alone / by
Loren W. Christensen
        p. cm.
    Includes index.
    ISBN 9781594394881
    1. Martial arts training -- Training. I. Title.

GV1102.7 T7 C455 2001
    769.8--dc21   2016909513

The author and publisher of the material are NOT RESPONSIBLE in any manner whatsoever for any injury that may occur through reading or following the instructions in this manual.

The activities, physical or otherwise, described in this manual may be too strenuous or dangerous for some people, and the reader(s) should consult a physician before engaging in them.

Warning: While self-defense is legal, fighting is illegal. If you don't know the difference, you'll go to jail because you aren't defending yourself. You are fighting—or worse. Readers are encouraged to be aware of all appropriate local and national laws relating to self-defense, reasonable force, and the use of weaponry, and act in accordance with all applicable laws at all times. Understand that while legal definitions and interpretations are generally uniform, there are small—but very important—differences from state to state and even city to city. To stay out of jail, you need to know these differences. Neither the author nor the publisher assumes any responsibility for the use or misuse of information contained in this book.

Nothing in this document constitutes a legal opinion, nor should any of its contents be treated as such. While the author believes everything herein is accurate, any questions regarding specific self-defense situations, legal liability, and/or interpretation of federal, state, or local laws should always be addressed by an attorney at law.

When it comes to martial arts, self-defense, and related topics, no text, no matter how well written, can substitute for professional, hands-on instruction. **These materials should be used for academic study only.**

Printed in USA

Contents

Using This Book

Throughout Solo Training, you will find icons that highlight important sections:

Sometimes you need to take extra care during your training. The caution symbol calls your attention to these places in the text.

Get the most out of every workout by paying special attention to these workout tips.

Advice you don't want to miss. Dsicovering the reasons behind the drills is just as important as doing the reps.

Although this is designed to be a book about training alone, some drills can be done with a partner. When you see this symbol, call up a friend!

Streamline your training for maximum impact with these expert training tips.

Introduction

I was 19 years old when I began studying karate in Portland, Oregon, and I fell in love with it the first time I saw that room full of people dressed in their white 'jammies', kicking and punching like a chorus line of dancers gone mad. I joined that night and quickly became one of the mad ones, devouring all the goodies like a chocolate lover in a candy store.

In the beginning, I had a hard time with the kicks because I was recuperating from a spinal injury I had suffered months earlier in a power lifting contest. The doctors told me to quit lifting and to find something else to do with my youthful energy that was less strenuous, like checkers or stamp collecting. It was 1965, and I, along with most of America, was uninformed as to what the martial arts were all about. I had heard something about karate, so I thought that it might be an easy-on-my-back way to burn some calories. Naive, huh?

That first class taught me how to rotate my hand when doing something called a "reverse punch" and how to sit in a.... a what? A horse stance? When the session was over, I was pleased to find that my back had survived, but that second class was a different story. That was when we were introduced to the front kick, and man oh man, did it ever hurt my lower back. Not only were my injured spine and damaged nerves rebelling against lifting my legs, but the tight adhesions that had formed over the injury prevented me from kicking higher than a short person's knee cap. I wasn't sure what I was going to do. After two lessons, I was already in love with karate and there was no way I could give it up before I had even started.

I decided to work on the problem at home. I held onto the back of a kitchen chair and swung my leg slowly forward and back, like an ancient, creaking pendulum. It made for some serious sweat-producing pain, but each day I trained at home, my leg went an inch or two higher to the front and a tad higher behind me. In class, I continued learning new material, which I did as well as I could. But at home and at my own pace, I pushed to break down the adhesions and work through the pain. Within a few weeks, I was able to kick as well as the other new students.

My instructor had not been sensitive to my problem and had been too busy with the huge school to give me special attention. If it had not trained alone at home, where I worked specifically on what I needed to work on, I would have never progressed. In fact, I would have probably dropped out because of my inability to do the techniques.

Although I initially trained alone to work through my injury, I discovered I enjoyed those workouts and began doing them regularly. I still lived with my parents then, and my mother complained that I was killing the grass in the backyard where I trained virtually every day. I also worked out in my bedroom, kicking at my bed post and standing along the wall trying to snap my punch out and back so fast that my fist wouldn't make a shadow. "What the heck are you doing in there?" my dad would call out at 2:00 a.m. when my snapping kicks and punches would awaken him.

For the next two years I enjoyed many wonderful workouts training alone. I continued to train in the backyard and in my bedroom, but I discovered other places, too. The garage, which had a dirt floor then, was dark and dank, but I trained in it anyway. I trained in my buddy's basement, as he slept away in another room, and I trained in the country under towering fir trees.

In the summer of 1967, I got a letter from Uncle Sam that read (after you cut through all the government-speak), "We want you in the 'Nam, boy." A month later I was off to the army. Boot camp and military police school were so intense that there was no time for karate training, though I did get a little hand-to-hand and judo training as part of the curriculum. But in my next four stops, K-9 school in Texas, security dog patrol duty in the Florida Everglades, Vietnamese language school in Washington, D.C. and police duty in the Vietnam, I managed to train alone and sometimes with the occasional training partner. I even attended a regular karate class for a while.

I shared a room with another soldier in Texas, but I was able to train alone when he was out drinking. In Florida, I attended a Japanese karate school in Miami, but when I trained alone in the Everglades, it was either in my room or behind the barracks, always vigilant for scorpions, snakes and 'gators. In Washington, D.C., I trained with a member of the army's elite fighting force, the Green Berets. I also trained alone in my room, though it measured only 10 by 12 feet, which didn't allow for a lot of training space with the bed and night stand. So I got inventive—when I practiced kicks, I raised the window and launched my foot out the opening (which must have looked rather strange from the ground). In my job as a military policeman in Vietnam, I had so much practical application of my techniques that I hardly needed practice. When I did, I would do it in an empty room or on a dusty road out in the boonies.

I consider these experiences, which went from 1965 to 1970, to be my formative years in the martial arts. They were to instill in me the value of training alone, something that has remained throughout the decades of my learning and teaching the martial arts. I'm convinced that 1/4 of the skill I've developed over the years, and 3/4 of the knowledge I have learned about myself, are a result of my spending time alone with my fighting art.

Although, I've always stressed training alone to my students, I'm not so naive to think that they all take my advice, though it's always obvious to me who does. For example, sometimes I'll suggest to a student that he work by himself on a special problem he is having or on something that he wants to improve, and within just two weeks, I can see whether he followed my advice. I especially delight in those times when I notice that a student's basic techniques, sparring, jujitsu, or arnis suddenly looks dramatically better than it did three weeks prior. "What have you been doing?" I ask, though I already know the answer.

The student usually blushes happily, and says, "You always say for us to train by ourselves, so I've been training a couple of extra days at home. I think it's really helped."

"Well, I *know* it has," I say. "Already there is a definite improvement."

Just as I have always encouraged my students to train alone, I want to encourage you to do the same. Those few minutes, just once or twice a week, that you devote to your fighting art outside of your normal class training, will give you returns on your effort many times over. Training alone will increase your knowledge of your fighting art's concepts, principles and techniques, and greatly increase your awareness of your inner strengths and weaknesses and physical strengths and weaknesses.

My purpose in writing *Solo Training* was not to replace your regular class instruction, but rather give you a valuable training concept that complements what your teacher is giving you. My intention was to not only cram the book with lots of training ideas that you can do by yourself when you can't make it to class, or when you want to train extra on material specific to your needs, but also to introduce you to some things that might be new to you.

There is nothing engraved in stone here, so feel free to modify the material as you see fit. If you cannot do something because of a physical limitation, teach it to someone else who might benefit. If you find something here that does not appeal to you, at least give it a try before you discard it. You just might be surprised and discover that it's the one thing that you have been looking for. Analyze the material to see how you can apply it to your particular fighting system, whether it's karate, kung fu, taekwondo, or whatever. If there is a technique or exercise that contradicts the way your style does it, but you find that you like the way it works, use it. Hey, I won't tell anyone in your school if you don't.

In closing this Introduction, let me encourage you to be creative in your training and to always question what you hear and read. I made the mistake in my early years of accepting blindly everything I was taught. That cost me a lot of time in my training.

A WORD ON THE WRITING

I use the word "karate" in the book as a generic way to refer to all the kick/punch arts: karate, taekwondo, kung fu and so on. I use "he" instead of the awkward he/she. I hope no one is offended by these writing techniques.

Warming Up

1

I know a champion fighter whose idea of warming up prior to a hard sparring session is to shake his legs a little and shrug his shoulders a couple times, if he does anything at all. Most of the time he just jumps right into the fray as soon as he ties on his belt. Does this mean that it's okay not to warm up? It definitely does not. My friend has just been lucky so far. One of these days, a cold muscle is going to go "Twang!" sending him to the sidelines for several months.

Keep in mind that your body may not be telling your brain the truth. Your legs, back and shoulders may feel loose and ready, especially on warm summer days, but it's still vitally important that you thoroughly warm up before you begin stressing your muscles, tendons and joints with kicks, punches and leaps. That readiness you feel as you change out of your street clothes into your training gear is a mix of enthusiasm and adrenaline. Don't let that fool you into believing that your body is ready. It isn't.

A proper warm up extends your endurance, prevents injuries and helps you achieve your training objective.

BUILD YOUR ENDURANCE

If you have ever warmed up by simply shaking your legs and shrugging your shoulders a couple of times, and then jumped right into a wild sparring session, you probably found yourself gasping for wind a few minutes later. The reason? You didn't properly prepare your heart, that all-important muscle that pumps oxygenated blood to all your moving parts. When your heart is included in your warm up, you are better prepared for the aerobic stress of sparring or vigorous kata.

WARD OFF INJURIES

Important

When all your body parts are well lubricated and moving smoothly from your warm up, you dramatically reduce the chance of injury. Think of your cold muscles, tendons and ligaments as being fragile as glass, and when you put excessive strain on them, they are at risk of breaking.

Your warm up needs to elevate your internal temperature a few degrees, elevate your pulse and respiration rate and get all your moving parts well lubricated. Even when you have reached this state, you should still hold off for a few minutes from doing those super-low stances and throwing kicks and punches that require hard snapping. Don't think of this as babying yourself or as not being macho. Think of it as training smart. There is no such thing as a Joints and Tendons are Us store where you can get replacements.

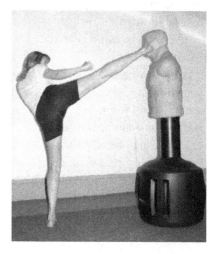

That rip you feel in your hamstring muscle is nature's way of saying that you should have warmed up more before throwing high kicks.

ACHIEVE YOUR GOALS

When your body is properly warmed and lubricated in preparation for your training, your techniques will flow more smoothly and be faster and stronger. The better you move, the more you improve. But when your muscles are cold, you move stiffly and awkwardly and improvement slows or doesn't occur at all.

THE MEDITATION WARM UP

I'm a firm believer in meditation, but I don't like doing it in the traditional seiza posture, that position where you kneel onto your knees and sit back on your heels. I've been in some schools where it's done after the warm-up and prior to the drills. The instructor tells the students to assume the sitting posture, close their eyes and have a moment of silence to prepare their brains for the learning that is to follow. This is all good and fine until the students have to get to their feet and begin a hard kicking drill. Their legs are stiff, maybe asleep and the kicks hurt for a few reps. Even the strict traditionalists know that this is risky to legs. Aikido teacher, Gakku Homma, says in his book *Aikido for Life*, "If you sit in seiza for a long time, your feet will go to sleep, so you cannot get up and move around easily for a while."

Don't use seiza as part of your warm up, because you are not warming anything at all. In fact, you are cutting off blood circulation to the lower half of your body. It's best to sit in meditation before your warm-up.

Caution

TWO WARM UPS

Here are two good methods to warm up. They are both effective, so choose one you like, or do a different one each workout.

Warm-up 1

This is a basic 8-minute warm-up that does a good job of preparing the body for training.

1. Shuffle around on the balls of your feet, rolling your shoulders and circling your arms. *2 minutes*

2. Do shoulder lifts, arm swings, easy punches, easy knee lifts and trunk twists. *2 minutes*

3. Swing your straight leg to the front, side and rear.
   1 set, 10 reps –each leg in each direction, 2 minutes

4. Easy roundhouse kicks, front kicks, side kicks and back kicks.
   1 set, 10 reps – each kick, each leg, 2 minutes

Warm-up 2

I have been using this warm up for about six months now in my class and when training alone. It's a fairly quick way to prepare for training, and it does a thorough job.

1. Arm loosening: rotate arms forward and backward.
   1 set, 10 reps – both arms, each direction

2. Good mornings: Place your hands behind your head, bend forward until your upper body is parallel with the floor and then return to the upright position.
   1 set, 15 reps

3. Side bends: Spread your feet and stretch your arms over your head. Bend as far as you can to the sides.
   1 set, 15 reps in each direction

4. Side-straddle hop (jumping jacks)
   1 set, 15 reps

5. Knee rotations: Place your knees together and rest your hands
   on them. Rotate your knees in each direction.
   1 set, 15 reps -- each direction

6. Dynamic leg stretching: this is a combination of lifting and
   swinging your straight leg upward. If you do it too slowly, it
   takes too much muscle action, which is not what you want. If
   you do it too fast, you could injure yourself. Your objective is to
   swing your legs a little higher on each rep.

   Important

   Front: Hold onto a wall or chair back and swing your
   straight leg up in front of you
   1 set, 10 reps – both legs

   Side: Face the wall or chair and swing your straight leg up
   to the side. Hold your foot in a side kick position
   1 set, 10 reps – both legs

   Rear curl: Face the wall or chair back and swing your leg
   back. When it's at its highest point, curl your lower leg as if
   trying to kick your rear.
   1 set, 10 reps – each leg

7. Chamber: Face the wall or chair back and swing your chambered leg up as if preparing to side kick or roundhouse. If the
   chambers for these two kicks are completely different in your
   style, do one method of chambering this workout and do the
   other method the next time you train alone.
   1 set, 10 reps – each leg.

   That is all there is to it. You can add reps as needed, but I
wouldn't advise doing any less than what is noted here. It's still a
good idea after completing this warm up to go easy the first few
minutes of your training.

COOL-DOWN

Important

Cooling down at the conclusion of your workout is just as important as the warm up, though it's most often neglected. When you have survived a 60 minute grueling solo workout, you just want to hit the shower and crash on the sofa. Spending another five or ten minutes doing cool down exercises is the last thing you feel like doing. But it's most important that you do because cooling down releases lactic acid that gathers in the muscles during a hard training session, which reduces that post workout stiffness and soreness.

Cool-down Exercises

Lightly stretch your legs, shoulders and arms for five to ten minutes at the completion of your workout. Use the same stretches you did to warm up your muscles and the same set and rep count, but do them with less intensity. Remember that you are cooling *down*.

Warm up properly, train safely and cool down properly and you will have many healthy, injury-free years in the martial arts.

2

Kicking

In this section we are going to explore ways to improve your kicking that are fun and innovative. We will look at how you can train alone to strengthen a weak kick, quickly improve a new one and explore ways to even increase the speed, power and flexibility in kicks you have been doing for a long time. We will also look at a few unusual kicks to see how you can use them in the street and in competition. As always, let's begin with the basics.

VARIATIONS OF THE BASIC KICKS

Let's begin with the basic four: front, round, side and back. These are the foundation of all leg techniques, which you must master before you can expect to perfect other ways of kicking. In addition, it's the front, round, side and back kicks that trained fighters commonly rely on in a self-defense situation. Hopefully, no one thinks they are going to use a leaping, spinning, cartwheel kick against a 245-pound ex-con who has spent the last ten years pumping iron in the joint and fighting other cons. Most martial artists who have fought in the street say that it was their fast and powerful basics that saved their bacon, not those fancy ones seen in silly movies.

A good way to thoroughly understand your basic kicks is to analyze the many ways they can be executed. Contrary to what you may have been told, the way that your school teaches the round-house, side kick, front kick and back kick is not the only way the basic kicks can be done. I mention this because there are narrow-minded styles and systems that teach that their way is the only way. This is nonsense. While there are certainly many ways to execute these kicks incorrectly, such as with poor balance, improper body mechanics, wrong angles and so on, there are many varied ways to execute them correctly. Not only are there variations among styles and systems, there are often variations found within the same fighting art.

I don't see a problem with this. What I do have a problem with are teachers who insist that their students kick exactly as they do. How can they expect this? How can a short-legged, broad-hipped student kick the same way as one who is long-legged and narrow-hipped? He cannot, nor should he be pushed to do so.

Training Tip

I first show my students the track of a kick. For example, I show them how a side kick is chambered, launched, extended, hits the target, retracted and returned to the floor. Once I see that they have the basic track, I let them discover how best to deliver it based on their physical structure. My job as the teacher is to ensure that they are employing the proper body mechanics, as they relate to their physique, to optimize their speed and power.

I also think it's important to examine other ways to execute the same kick. We are blessed with a melting pot of styles and systems in this country, so we should take advantage and borrow and steal from each other. If you are a kung fu fighter but you really like taekwondo's roundhouse kick, why shouldn't you add it to your repertoire?

If you belong to a strict system that doesn't allow for variations, I leave that to you to work it out with your teacher. I'm not suggesting that you be disrespectful or a traitor to your school, but if your teacher is unbendable, you have to decide if a rule is more important than a technique that may save your life. I've used my fighting art on the streets in Vietnam and as a cop in Portland, Oregon, so that decision has never been a tough one for me.

In this section, let's take a look at a few variations of the front, round, back and side kicks. We will examine different parts of your foot and leg to kick with, as well as different ways to launch the kick. These kicking methods may be different from the way you regularly do them, so training alone is the perfect time to experiment, especially if your school has a strict policy as to how kicks are to be performed. Practice them away from your school and then use them on your classmates. When your kick smacks into them and they are left standing there scratching their heads, saying, "What the heck was that?" it will be interesting to hear their arguments against the technique.

Front KICK

The front kick, with the front or rear leg, is often the first kick taught to beginning students, though that doesn't make it the easiest one to learn. Even an untrained person can do a kick that looks like a front kick, but to do it properly takes a lot of work. It's important that you know how the body mechanics of the front thrust kick are different from those that make up the front snap kick. I'm not going to take the space here to describe them because every other book on the market does a good job of it. Just make sure you have a good understanding of the differences before you proceed to the variations that follow.

Angle Front Kick

This is one of my favorite front kicks because it's so deceptive. It launches forward at an angle, half way between a straight front kick and a circular roundhouse kick. To do it, simply angle your lower leg out slightly—use your fast front leg or your more powerful rear leg, depending on which element you need at the time—and kick forward into the target. Kick with the ball of your foot, the top of your foot or your lower shin, just above your ankle. The difference depends on the target. For instance, if you are kicking an assailant's thigh, hit with the ball of your foot. Kick him with the top of your foot, however, if you are firing at his groin or at his face as he is bent over looking downward.

A nice feature of the angle front kick is that an assailant can be turned three quarters away from you, but the angle of your kick allows your foot to "sneak" around his upper thigh and whack him in the groin.

3 sets, 15 reps — both front legs
3 sets, 15 reps — both rear legs

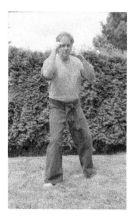

From your on-guard position (1), lift your leg into a slanted chamber(2) and launch the angled front kick (3).

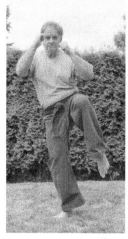

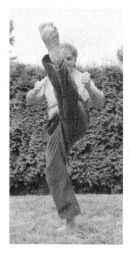

Push Kick

This is an important kick that I never considered until I began watching full-contact fighters, especially Muay Thai competitors. As the name implies, the kick is a pushing action as opposed to a thrusting one. Although it can hurt your opponent, it's mostly used to keep him off you or to set him up for a second technique. If you are quick and your opponent is slow, the push kick can be used to jam his hip as he chambers it.

Kick with the entire bottom of your foot or with just the ball. Use the bottom if you just want to push your opponent away or to stop him from advancing on you. If you have time to add a shot of pain to the push, use the ball of your foot and aim at his groin, thigh, or knee. You can use your rear foot, though most full-contact fighters use the lead since it's closer and quicker. When using the front leg, shift your weight to your rear leg, bend your rear knee a little and push your front leg into the target. If you want to move forward as you push, move your rear foot up to the heel of your lead foot and then execute the push kick with your front leg.

Practice against a swinging heavy bag. As it comes towards you, push it away.

3 sets, 10 reps — each leg

Upside Down Front Kick

I learned this weird kick years ago from a kajukenbo fighter. He called it "cobra kick," which is fairly descriptive as to how it looks when it strikes an opponent in the face or chest. I doubt its usefulness as a street technique, but it's fun to sneak in when sparring and when practicing drills with a partner. Besides being a tricky kick, it's a great exercise because it works the front kick muscles at a different angle. Here is how you do it.

Get in a left-leg-forward fighting stance. To chamber the kick, flip your lower, left leg outward while keeping your knee pointing downward (the position of your knee makes it difficult for an opponent to counter kick you to the groin). The chamber is complete when your foot, which is tucked as close to your rear as you can get it, is upside down and pointing at the target. To kick, simply thrust the ball of your foot into the target.

Air: 3 sets, 15 reps – both sides

Applying broken rhythm: Here is how you can use broken rhythm to set it up ("Broken Rhythm," page 165). Throw two or three lead-leg roundhouses at your opponent, allowing him to block them. This establishes a rhythm and an expectation in his mind that when he sees your leg chamber, you are going to throw a circular kick. The next time, bring your chamber up as if you were going to roundhouse kick, but continue to swing your lower leg up until your knee is pointing downward and the bottom of your kicking foot is pointing at the ceiling. Since you have established an expectation in him, he will probably begin to block outward toward what he thinks is going to be a roundhouse. But you are too tricky and thrust your upside down front kick on a straight line right into his breadbasket.

Air: 3 sets, 15 reps –both sides

When escaping: It also works great when moving away from an opponent. Assume a left-leg- forward fighting stance. As your opponent moves toward you, retreat in your usual fashion by moving your right foot back to your left and then moving your left foot back. The next time he advances, do it again, establishing a rhythm in his mind. The third time he comes in, lean back to create an illusion that you are again moving away, but when he is in range, fire the kick in for the score. Ha,ha.

Air: 3 sets, 10 reps – both sides

Practice the upside down front kick in the air and on the bag. It's a deceptive kick when sparring and, as an exercise, it's a fun break from pounding out rep after rep of the standard front kick.

Heavy bag: 3 sets, 15 reps – both sides

Seated Front Kicks

Workout
Tip

Practicing your front kicks while seated is a good exercise as well as an excellent offensive move that you should know how to do. As an exercise, it places a great deal of stress on your upper thigh and hip because you cannot lean back when throwing the kick. As an offensive or defensive technique, front kicking from a seated position can be quite surprising to an assailant.

Sit in an armless chair and grab the sides of your seat (the chair's seat, not yours). Slowly chamber your front kick and extend your leg as high as you are able. Hold it there for a second and take masochistic joy in the burning and knotting sensation that is happening in your leg muscles. Rechamber and return your foot to the floor. Do slow reps to develop strength, and fast reps to work your fast twitch muscles.

Slow reps: 1 set, 10 reps — each leg
Fast reps: 2 set, 10 reps — each leg

Extra credit: Make up a few self-defense scenarios and see what you can and cannot do from the chair. For example, block an imaginary attacker's punch, front kick him, get to your feet quickly and finish him off. Consider grabbing the back of the chair and using it to block and hit with.

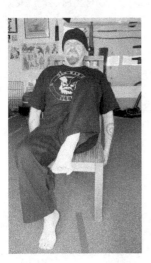

Hold onto the sides of the chair's seat and chamber your front kick. Extend your kick as high as you are able and hold it for one second.

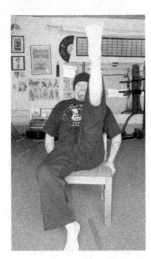

Squat Kicks

If you want to know which muscles this exercise affects, do several sets of high reps your first time and see if you can get out of bed the next day. If you manage to get up, the front of your thighs and knees will scream and buckle with your every step. For sure, this exercise gets right to heart of the front kick and, when done systematically, will help develop explosiveness. Here is how you do it.

Keep both arms in an on-guard position and your feet together as you squat down until your thighs are parallel with the floor. Now, drive yourself up as fast as you are able and launch a left front kick. Immediately snap it back and drop back down into your low squat. Spring right back up again, but this time launch a right front kick. Immediately snap it back and return to your deep squat. Be sure to keep your back straight throughout your reps and be cautious not to bounce at the bottom of the squat as this defeats the purpose of the exercise and can injure your knees.

Caution

Two variations:

1. To work on strength and explosiveness, push yourself up fast, kick fast, but lower yourself slowly back to the squat.
2. If you want to train for endurance and explosiveness, do as many reps as you can in 60 seconds, alternating your legs each kick.

Be kind to yourself with this exercise and don't overdo it your first workout. Even if you are in good condition, it's a good idea to start with one set and progress slowly over several weeks to three sets.

For strength and explosiveness: *1-3 sets, 10 reps — each leg.*
For endurance and explosiveness: *1-3 sets, 60 seconds each —alternating each leg.*

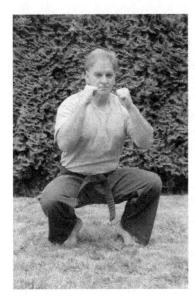

Hold both of your arms in an on-guard position and drive yourself up as fast as you can and execute a front kick.

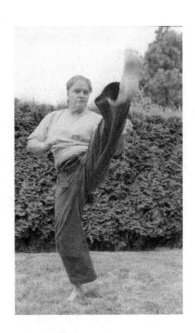

Kneeling Front Kick

This is similar to the last exercise, though most people find it more of a challenge. Eat the pain and you will develop incredible leg power.

Kneel on the floor with your knees in front of you as you sit back on your heels. If you can't sit all the way back, go as far as you can. If it hurts one or both knees, you may not want to do the exercise at all because it only gets worse from this point on. Thrust your right leg forward and throw a left reverse punch. As you retract your punch, throw a left-leg front kick as high as you can (it probably won't be too high), while coming up off your right knee only enough to allow your kicking foot to clear the floor. Retract your kick until your knee is again on the floor, and then drop your right knee and sit back on your heels. That is one rep. You got lots more to do.

The punch is an extra added element in case you need to get in some punching during your workout. I like to include it because it gets me thinking about my energy moving forward, and it feels more like I'm doing a self-defense drill rather than an exercise. If it confuses you at first, take it out of the exercise and do only the kicks. Add it later when you feel you are ready to do more.

2 sets, 10 reps — each side

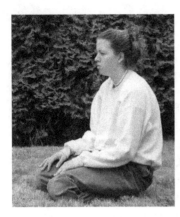

Begin in a kneeling position. Thrust your right leg forward and execute a left reverse punch.

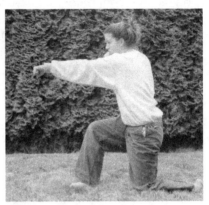

As you retract your punch, throw a left-legged front kick and then drop back to the one-leg-up kneeling position and then all the way back to the both-knees-down starting position.

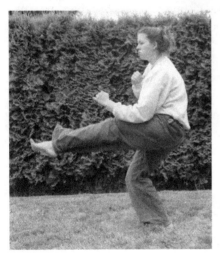

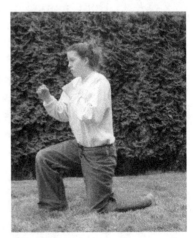

BACK KICK

The back kick is arguably the strongest kick in the martial arts, its power driven by the large gluteus maximus (butt) muscles. I can tell you from experience, it's the best kick for smashing in doors on drug houses, even those that have been reinforced on the inside.

There are two versions of the standing back kick: lead-leg and turning. When you have your left leg forward, execute a lead-leg back kick by turning your upper body to the right and then thrusting your *left* foot straight into the target. To execute a turning back kick, turn your upper body to the right and thrust your *right* foot into the target. Always look over the shoulder of the side that is kicking. Most styles execute the kick the same way, although some traditionalist chamber the knee in front while others simply launch the kicking foot straight from the floor. My preference is to kick from the floor because it saves time. Any loss of power by not chambering is negligible.

No matter how you launch the two versions, here are a few important points to watch out for when practicing alone:

Training Tip

Hit with the heel. Making contact with the toes or the ball of the foot is a sure way to get an injury.

Don't look over your opposite shoulder when kicking as the severe twist may injure your spine.

Don't "unwind" your body (returning to your original position) after you have executed a turning back kick. Instead, kick and drop your foot to the floor in front of you.

Make sure the trajectory is straight out from your rear, as opposed to turning too far and making the kick a turning side kick.

Don't hook your leg on the return, as you do when roundhouse kicking.

Don't lean too far away from the target. The impact will be reduced and it will knock you off balance.

Here are a few ways to practice the two basic back kicks by yourself to help improve your accuracy.

Kick at a spot on the wall (as shown in *Fighter's Fact Book*)
Kick at your image in a mirror
Kick at a mark on a heavy bag
Kick at an object hanging from the ceiling: ball, wad of paper, rolled sock, hacky-sack, etc

Here are some fun and practical variations on the back kick. As with any new technique, especially those that are sensitive to balance, they might require a little extra work so that you don't fall into a heap.

Touch Back Kick

This is an interesting back kick that is easier to do than it looks. Even if you are not flexible, you can kick chest high, even head high because of the way in which your body is aligned. Unless you are especially fast with it, you shouldn't use it as a lead attack since you have to turn your back on your opponent and drop down into a relative precarious position to kick. It works especially well, however, when in the course of a fight your back is to the opponent and you are falling. It's also effective when you are on the ground and your opponent rushes you.

Here are a few variations of the touch back kick. Be careful of the standing ones because even though the kick doesn't require a great deal of flexibility, you can still strain your support leg. As an added caution, be careful the first few times you do the standing touch-back kick against a live opponent. Both of you will be surprise when your foot shoots up higher than you intended and your heel crunches your partner's chin.

Lead-leg, Touch Back Kick

Stand before a mirror and square off against your image with your left foot forward. Snap your body hard to the right while angling it downward, touch the floor with your right hand and kick back with your left leg. Look along your left side to see the target.

From your left-leg-forward, on-guard position, turn to your right, lean down and touch the floor with your right hand and kick upward with your left leg.

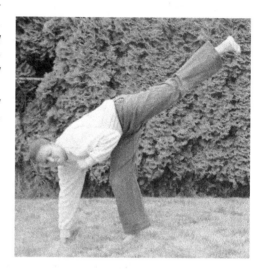

Turning Touch Back Kick

Square off against your image in the mirror with your left leg forward. Although you should be looking in the area of your opponent's chin, for the sake of developing accuracy, look at and aim for the center of your chest in the mirror. Turn the same way you do when executing a turning back kick, but as you turn, angle your upper body to the floor and touch it with one or both hands.

3 sets, 10 reps – both sides

On One Knee

Say you are on the ground, right knee down and left knee up, when the assailant advances on you from your front. Pivot hard away from him to your right as you pivot around on your right knee (your lower right leg will turn to the right, too). Touch the floor with both hands and kick upward with your left leg. Don't expect to kick as high as you do when standing. Look along your left side to see the target, such as a mark on the wall.

3 sets of 10 reps — each side

Back Kick for Flexibility and Power

This two-part exercise will put stretch in your back kick, power in the muscles and build buns of steel. Yesss!

For flexibility   Let's begin with the stretch. Grab hold of a support and swing your right leg up behind you as high as you are able. Keep your leg stiff, lead with your heel and lean your upper body forward no more than 45 degrees.

1 set, 20 reps -- each leg

After you have completed one stretching set with each leg, move to the power-building portion of the exercise.

For power   Hold onto your support as before and lift your leg up behind you, leading with your heel. This time, lift your leg slowly so that it's muscle lifting your leg, not momentum. You won't be able to go as high as you did with the flexibility phase, and that is okay. When you have reached your highest point, hold your leg in that position for 10 to 15 seconds without bending your upper body more than 45 degrees. If you get a knot in your butt, lower your leg, shake it out and continue with the next rep.

Workout
Tip

1 set, 10-15 reps — each leg

BASIC SIDE KICK

There are at least two methods to side kick that are considered basic: the snap version and the thrust. The snap kick uses the knee joint as a hinge to flip out the lower leg. I think snapping takes its toll on the knee joint, so much so that it might shorten the training careers of some fighters who have vulnerable knees to begin with. The problem is that they don't always know they have vulnerable knees until they begin having problems. In some cases, that may be too late.

There are fighters who can do beautiful, high snap kicks, even over their opponents' heads. But hey can't hit the heavy bag hard with it. If your high snap kick is only for kata or demonstrations, you have to decide whether you want to pound the bag with it. But if you consider it a weapon for self-defense, you absolutely need to work with it on the heavy bag to know that you can deliver it with sufficient power to hurt or at least stop an assailant.

I only do snap side kicks to the shin and knee because my knees and hips complain bitterly when I try to snap higher. I use thrust side kicks for all targets higher than my opponent's shins. A thrust might take a hair of a second longer to get to the target, but it's much easier on the knees and causes much more damage to the target.

A police war story: I had a workout partner many years ago who was a cop and a black belt. He was a powerful guy, though slender, with a thrust side kick that could send a rhino rolling. One night a big drunk discovered this for himself when he burst out the back of the paddy wagon and rushed my friend. That thrust side kick of his nailed the drunk right under the armpit and literally lifted him in the air, just like those fake photos on the cover of karate magazines. But the drunk was flying for real, about two feet off the pavement and backwards until he slammed painfully into the side of the paddy wagon. He sort of stuck there for a second and then began to crumple, like the Roadrunner in the cartoon does after he hits the side of a mountain. The big drunk slid down the side of the wagon and onto his butt, where he sat for several minutes listening to little chirping birds all about his fuzzy head.

Two Basic Methods of Chambering and Kicking

Some people launch their side kicks by first bringing their kicking knees straight up in front of their bodies, as if they were chambering a front kick. When their knees have reached the desired height, they snap their hips around and launch their side kicks. Although it's a variation used by several champions, I have had many students complain that it hurts their knee joints after a few repetitions.

Perhaps the most common method to side kick is for the kicker to position the side of his body toward the target, chamber his leg as high as he can and then thrust. This is a powerful version, though not as fast as snapping it out. The weakness with it is that you have to turn your body to the side, which takes time and can telegraph your intent if you don't camouflage your movements.

Important

Since this is the most common way to side kick, let's see how you can hide your intention to kick.

Shuffle to Camouflage your Setup

If you are like most fighters, you probably fight with your body angled a quarter turn away from your opponent. This means you have to deliberately turn your body one extra quarter turn to the side to launch the side kick, a movement that takes time and announces your intent. Here is a way to camouflage your setup.

When sparring, keep your body in motion by twisting your lead foot, as if positioning it for a side kick, and making short, snapping movements with your upper body toward the side stance. Repeating these actions two or three times without actually kicking conditions your opponent to seeing them but not to expect anything further. Then when you really do follow through with a side kick, it takes him a second or two to realize that you are doing more than just that weird twisting thing. A second is all the time you need to nail him with the kick.

Practice camouflaging your set up in front of a mirror.

3 sets, 10 reps – both sides

Side-to-side shuffle This variation of shuffling to camouflage your side kick looks a little strange, but it works. Assume your left-leg-forward fighting stance. As you move about stalking your imaginary opponent, hide your intention to side kick by moving your left foot over to your right about two feet, as if you were going to hook kick from the floor, and then swing your foot back to your left about two feet, all the while maintaining contact with the floor. Repeat this three or four times to confuse your opponent so that he doesn't know if you are preparing to throw a hook kick or a roundhouse. Ha! It's neither. Right in the middle of that shuffle, when he is at his most confused, thrust your side kick into his ribs.

3 sets, 10 reps – both sides

Side Kick Check

This variation of the side kick is not meant to hurt the assailant (but that is okay if it does), but is used more to keep him and his buddies away from you, similar to the way a boxer uses his jab. Since you are not delivering a full-power strike, you need only a minimum chamber before you snap out your kick to his shin or knee, and then snap it back. Always hit with the heel half of your foot since it's the strongest and is supported by your lower leg.

Consider using the side kick check when facing two or more assailants, especially the types who don't charge straight in but hop in and out of range as they punch and kick at you. Right after you punch that one on the right, snap a fast side kick check to the shin of that guy coming at you from the left. The kick will either cause him to jump back, or at least distract him briefly, giving you time to follow up.

To practice this, set a heavy bag on the floor in the corner of your room and begin shadow sparring around it. Imagine an assailant stepping toward you and you stop him with a quick side kick check to his shin (the bag). Afterwards, move quickly away or follow up with a couple of fast hand blows to the air over the bag. You can also practice by standing sideways to an imaginary assailant (the bag) in a neutral stance, as if waiting for a bus. Imagine that he suddenly steps threateningly into your space. Side kick check the bag at knee level and then step quickly away as if to flee, or turn and face the bag and execute follow up blows over the top of it.

Shadow spar: 10 minutes – execute an equal number of side kick checks with each leg

From neutral stance: 2 sets, 15 reps – both sides

Bent over Side Kick

When you are bent over at the waist, it's impossible to front kick and a roundhouse kick, though possible, is weak. You can, however, launch a strong side kick. Perhaps you are bent over because you just ate a hard kick to your stomach, or your assailant has you in an arm bar hold. Or maybe you are a tricky fighter and you are faking an injury so that your assailant relaxes his guard and moves into range. For whatever reason, your upper body is bent 90 degrees at the waist.

If your opponent has you in an arm bar, extend an arm out to your side to simulate the hold. Adjust your feet so that you are sideways to him and drive a side kick into his leg. If you are pretending to be bent as a result of a blow or you are trying to make him think you are hurt, adjust your angle so you are sideways to your imaginary target, and drive a side kick into his thigh, knee or shin. Both of these scenarios look a little odd when pantomiming by yourself, so make sure no one is looking in the window.

Arms extended out your sides: 2 sets, 10 reps — each leg
Bent as if struck: 2 sets, 10 reps — each leg

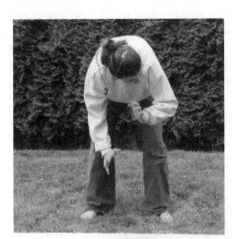

From a bent-over position, adjust your angle so you are sideways to your opponent. As quick as you can, drive a sidekick into his leg or hip.

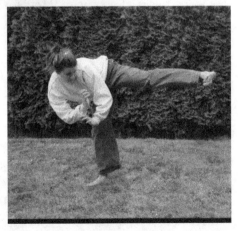

Side kick Exercises

These exercises not only build strength in the thrust portion of the kick, but also at the focus point, that place where your leg is extended and your foot is making contact with the target. These are not fun exercises, so don't expect to have a lot of laughs doing them. They are highly effective, though.

Side kick and hold   There are two variations to this exercise, one where you strive to increase the amount of time you hold your leg out, and the other where you push to increase the height of your kick. Both variations greatly improve your balance, muscle control, hip flexibility and all the muscles involved in your support leg. Here is how you do them:

Time: Slowly extend your side kick as high as you can with flawless form, and then hold it at full extension for 10 seconds per rep. Grit your teeth and fight to prevent your leg from sinking. Over the weeks, increase the time to 30 seconds per rep.
1 set, 10 reps, 10- 30-second each — each leg

Height: Slowly extend your leg as high as you can using your hip and leg power. When your leg is fully extended, take hold of your pant leg with your finger tips and pull your leg up as far as you can and hold it there. Be careful not to let your arms do all the work; this is a leg exercise. Hold for 5 seconds and then slowly chamber and return to the floor. That is one rep.
2 sets, 10, 5-second reps — each leg

Seated side kicks   Okay, enough fun. Here is one that will put a nice knot in your upper thigh and hip. It's a seated exercise, so it's hard to cheat by leaning excessively away from the direction that you are kicking in. The position places considerable strain on the muscles involved in the side kick, so much so that you have to keep telling yourself that this is good for you. Here is how you do it.

Sit in an armless chair and face forward. Lift your right knee in front of you and slowly extend it to the side in a perfect side kick. You can lean your upper body a little, but not too much since you want to make those side kick muscles work. Strive for precise form and for as much height as you can (which won't be very high) to really get a feel for how those muscles are working. Do slow reps to develop power and fast reps to stimulate your fast-twitch muscles.

Workout Tip

Slow chair side kicks: 1 set, 10 reps -- each leg
Fast chair side kicks: 1 set, 10 reps -- each leg

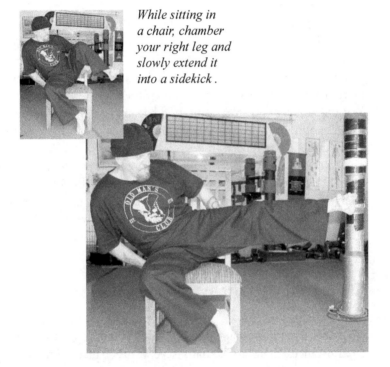

While sitting in a chair, chamber your right leg and slowly extend it into a sidekick.

Extra credit After you have trashed your muscles doing the chair exercises, finish your workout with this fun drill. The idea is to practice scenarios from your chair as you did with the front kick. Pretend that you are blocking a shoulder grab from the side and counter with a side kick. Leap to your feet and finish him off with whatever you choose. Have fun with it and learn what you can and cannot do while sitting.

THE BASIC ROUNDHOUSE KICK

Taekwondo fighters definitely don't throw their roundhouse kicks the same way Muay Thai fighters do. In fact, not all tae-kwondo and Muay Thai fighters throw their roundhouses in the same fashion. The same is true of the various Chinese, Japanese and American eclectic systems. They all have subtle, or not so subtle, variations that have developed over time either by deliberate intent or happenstance.

Is one method better than the other? Who knows for sure? To conduct a scientific study would be overwhelmingly complex because of the large number of variables that would have to be factored in. My advice is that you first master the method taught in your style and then examine how other styles perform theirs. You may or may not find a method so superior that you want to replace yours, but you probably will find one or more that you want to include in your repertoire.

I encourage you to examine your basic roundhouse kick to learn all the variations that are possible with it. Begin by asking yourself questions about it and then seek out the answers. For example, how can you deliver it faster? More powerfully? How can you better set up your roundhouse to successfully get it in on an opponent, both offensively and defensively?

Important

Kicking with All Parts of Your Leg

Perhaps you learned to roundhouse kick by making contact with only the top of your foot. This is fine, but depending on the circumstances there are actually several other places on your leg that you connect with. Use your solo time to experiment to see how versatile the roundhouse kick really is.

The Ball of the Foot

When I began training back in the 1960s, we learned to round-house kick barefoot with the ball of the foot, just as our teachers learned in the Orient. That was okay until I was in the military. On several occasions in Vietnam, I kicked people with the ball of my foot while wearing combat boots. I curled my toes back as I had done in class, but the heavy, steel-toed boot didn't curl, so every time I ended up limping afterwards with a sprained ankle and jammed toes. Since I'm a slow learner, I hurt myself several times before it dawned on me what I was doing wrong. When I changed to kicking with the shoestring area of my boot, the problem went away.

But don't let my experience discourage you from considering the ball of the foot as an impact point. Perhaps you wear really flexible shoes and you can kick with the ball of your foot while wearing them (they aren't those gold-colored ones that curl up on each end, are they?). Or maybe you train for other reasons than self-defense, so it doesn't matter to you that you can't curl your toes back in your street shoes.

To be completely confident kicking with the ball of the foot, I highly suggest that you practice on the heavy bag. Take it easy at first, because a bent-back toe is not a fun moment to live in. Although you can use the ball of the foot to kick any target, from your opponent's head to his shin, I think it's a big risk to kick someone in the head with it. If your foot is angled wrong, a jammed toe against someone's hard skull is going to send you spiraling to the floor, wailing like a newborn babe.

Caution

One of my black belts loves to kick with the ball of his foot to the inside of his opponent's thigh, and it really hurts. He doesn't stretch his leg out as he would if he were kicking to the head, but he keeps it bent and delivers it within punching range. Like a boxer with a quick jab, he pops his kick to that tender spot every time his opponent starts to move in on him. He knows it's doubtful that he could use it while wearing shoes, but he doesn't care because he is having too much fun putting little bruises on everyone's thighs.

Practice kicking the bag at all heights so you are familiar with how your foot position needs to be modified. But if you just want to kick at one height, say the abdomen or to mid thigh, concentrate your bag work at that level.

Heavy bag: 3 sets, 15 reps —each foot
Air: 3 sets, 15 reps — each foot

Shoestring Area

The most common impact point for the roundhouse kick is the top of the foot where your shoestrings are laced. Since it's a broad surface, it lacks the penetration that kicking with the ball-of-the-foot has, but it's safer on your toes. Should you kick someone in the point of his chin, you risk breaking the fine bones on the top of your foot, but it's relatively safe when kicking to non boney surfaces. Kicking with the top of the foot is effective in competition because it provides you with several inches of reach versus kicking with the ball.

Any target from the side of the face to the calf is good, but be cautious of kicking boney surfaces. The kidneys, ribs, groin and thighs are favorites because impact to them can cause debilitation.

Air: 3 sets, 15 reps — each leg.
Heavy bag: 3 sets, 15 reps — each leg

Lower Shin

Important

Muay Thai fighters believe so much in the effectiveness of kicking with their lower shin, that portion of the leg 6 to 10 inches above the ankle, that they use it almost exclusively to knock their opponents into Tweety Bird land. They believe that the foot is weak and that it lacks support. The shin, however, is a hard and thick bone that when slammed at 60 mph into a human target, the target loses.

If you haven't used the lower shin as an impact point, the hardest part of kicking with it is making the mental adjustment to do so. First, you have to implant the idea in your mind to use it. Secondly, you have to adjust your range from the target. Since you are kicking with an area that is higher up on your leg, you need to be about 12 inches closer to the target than when kicking with the top of your foot. Once the mental and physical adjustments are made, you will wonder why you didn't kick with your shin before.

Begin by thinking *shin* as you practice your reps in the air, and aim it at your imaginary target on each rep.

Air reps: 3 sets, 20 reps — each leg

If you have tender shins, wear your shin guards when kicking the heavy bag. With the added padding, you can slam it hard without screaming out in pain and hopping around on one leg.

Heavy bag: 3 sets, 20 reps —each leg

Roundhouse Knee

Moving up the leg (do I sound like a travel guide?), we come to the boney knee cap. First a warning. Have you ever bumped knees with your training partner? What a laugh riot, huh? It's for that painful reason that it's not a good idea to deliberately slam your knee cap against a boney surface on your opponent's body, such as his skull, knee, shin or elbow. You can get away with hitting a hard surface if you make impact a couple of inches above or below your knee, but if you hit with your knee cap, you may find yourself as out of commission as your opponent. To be safe, strike only soft targets on your opponent.

You can execute a roundhouse-knee strike with either your front or rear leg. The front is fastest, since it's closest to the target, and your rear leg is strongest since it's traveling the greatest distance and gets help from your hip rotation. To add power to the impact, grab your opponent's shoulders or the back of his neck, and pull him in hard as you drive your round knee into him. The direction follows the same circular track as your roundhouse kick. Pull his body forward, rotate your hips and drive your knee in hard. Rise up on the ball of your foot at the point of impact to deliver just a little more energy into the target. It's a great technique to slip under an opponent's arms or to drive into the side of his thigh.

Simulate grabbing with both your hands behind your imaginary opponent's neck to pull him toward you, and drive in your round knee.

Air reps: 3 sets, 15 reps — each knee

With the heavy bag, grab the top of it and pull toward you as you ram in your knee. Be sure to rotate your hips for maximum power.

Heavy bag: 3 sets, 15 reps — both knees

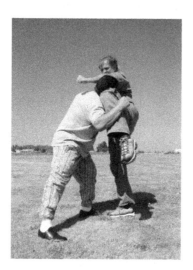

Training Tip

Kicking with the Thigh

Although this is seldom used, it's a great technique for punishing an attacker who tries to pull you in close for a clinch. The direction of force is circular and the striking area is your thigh, that place just above your knee to about mid-thigh. The leg is held the same as when executing the round knee strike, and the hips are rotated in the same fashion. Timing-wise, it works great when the two of you are about 12 inches apart and moving toward each other.

You need to fire it off quickly because once you are in the clinch, you are too close for the blow to have sufficient impact. Even when you are in the ideal range, the blow is not terribly powerful since your thigh doesn't travel far enough to build significant momentum. Nonetheless, it's still capable of whooshing the air out of your opponent when you drive it into his ribs, especially right under the bottom one, or make him dizzy when you hit him in the head. The impact can be increased by pulling your opponent into the blow.

Simulate holding onto your opponent and pull him into the blow.

Air reps: 3 sets, 15 reps — each side

Pull from the top of the heavy bag to simulate pulling your opponent into your kick. Be sure to bend you're your leg as you kick because driving your thigh into the bag with a straight leg may hyperextend your knee, which is in the Top 5 of things you can do to yourself that really, really hurt.

Heavy bag: 3 sets, 10 reps – both sides

Roundhouse Kick Exercises

Workout
Tip

Here are a couple of exercises that add power, speed and dexterity to all of your roundhouse kick variations.

Sacrifice roundhouse kick   I doubt the effectiveness of this concept in a real fight, but it's a fun trick to use in your school sparring and in competition. It develops flexibility, speed and power in your legs, so if you don't have those elements yet, don't try this technique against an opponent. Instead, use this as an exercise to develop those attributes. Spend time training alone on this and when you can do it quick as a wink, take it to your class and surprise your buddies with it.

The roundhouse kick is arguably the easiest offensive leg technique to do in karate, so much so that it's the most often used in class and in competition. It's easy to do, and it's also easy to block, even by students with just a couple of months training. And that is okay, because you are going to use that to your advantage.

Face the mirror with your left side forward. Step up with your rear foot and throw a roundhouse kick with your lead leg. Pretend that it was blocked and snap it back just far enough to change it to a side kick without your foot touching the floor. The switch is easy to do, but it takes training to do it with speed, which you need to get the side kick into the opening that was made by his roundhouse block.

Let's say you do the sacrifice roundhouse and you roll it nicely into the side kick. But your opponent is having a good day and blocks or jams your second kick, too. Instead of setting your leg down and cursing under your breath, roll your leg right back into a roundhouse chamber and pop another roundhouse into his ribs. Ha, ha on him. This works because you are kicking at different angles: You start with a circular kick, abruptly change it to a linear one and then back to a circular one. Your opponent's eyes will be rolling in their sockets like a cartoon character's.

To reiterate, if you don't have the flexibility, speed and strength right now to do this as well as you would like, don't worry about it. You will develop those attributes by doing repetitions, lots of them.

Here are a few other combinations using the roundhouse kick that are good exercises because they develop hip and leg strength, flexibility and the ability to change directions of force quickly. Be sure to do all the kicks before returning your foot to the floor. Work them hard as an exercise and soon you will be using them against an opponent.

Roundhouse kick, side kick, roundhouse kick
Roundhouse kick, front kick, roundhouse kick
Roundhouse kick low, roundhouse kick high
Roundhouse kick, hook kick, side kick
Roundhouse kick, side kick, hook kick
Air reps: 3 sets, 10 reps -- both sides, each combination

Superset roundhouse drill   This is a simple but effective two-part exercise I've been using since I read an article about it written by Black Belt Hall of Fame member Jon Valera in the March 2000 issue of "Martial arts Training" magazine. Though simple, it's a tough one that when done consistently will develop power, endurance and explosiveness in your roundhouse.

Part one: Assume a left-leg-forward fighting stance in front of a heavy, hanging bag. Whip a right roundhouse kick into the bag and then retract it all the way back to its starting position. Repeat for one minute and then switch your stance and kick with your other leg for one minute. Don't stroll in the park here, but go all out for as many reps as you can squeeze into 60 seconds.

Part two: Now, without pausing, you are ready for the second part of the superset: roundhouse kicking with the front leg. So that you begin this set with a relatively fresh right leg, assume a right-leg-forward fighting stance. Whip out as many hard and fast lead-leg roundhouse kicks as you are able in one minute. Switch stances and do the same with your left leg.

Here is how the superset looks:
Rear-leg roundhouse kicks: 1 set, 60 seconds —each leg
Front-leg roundhouse kicks: 1 set, 60 seconds —each leg

FIVE USEFUL KICKS

Free of charge, I'm including five of my favorite kicks that are sort of out of the norm but have always served me well. Although many fighting systems incorporate them, there are many more that don't. I encourage you to include them in your fighting repertoire because they are sneaky, versatile and they can be combined easily with other techniques to make effective combinations.

Here is how you do them and how you can practice them on your own.

Funny Kick

I learned this technique from a friend who studies and teaches kajukenbo, an eclectic system developed in the late 1940s by five instructors from five different arts, specifically, Korean karate, jujitsu, judo, kenpo and kung fu. The funny kick was designed by them because they wanted a fast, deceptive and hard-to-block kick that required little flexibility and could be delivered with minimum telegraphing. The funny kick does all this while looking sort of odd in the process.

This is because your foot moves toward the target on a circular path and connects with the *outside edge* (the little-toe side) of your foot.

Assume a left-leg-forward stance and make a sharp twist of your upper body to your right as you "flip out" your lower leg using the hinge action of your knee. The knee actually points down throughout the motion, which provides several advantages. Your upper leg is in the way, so your all-important groin is protected against your opponent's counter kick, which is not the case with the standard roundhouse that also travels on a circular path. There is a minimum of telegraphing since you don't have to lift the leg prior to kicking, which makes it an effective kick against strong counter punchers. Although the lack of telegraphing makes it a great kick for the street, it can be hard for tournament judges to see since the delivery is different than the usual roundhouse kick. Try shouting as you kick to draw their attention to it.

Important

It's also a good street technique because you can flip it easily into an assailant's groin even when you are wearing tight pants (I once tore the crotch out of my pants in a street scuffle when I threw a head-high roundhouse kick). Since the motion of the funny kick comes from the hinge action of your knee as opposed to body momentum, its impact is not as great as other kicks. While kicking an opponent in the stomach, chest or head will get you points in competition, it's doubtful it would stop an enraged person or a drug-sopped street creep. When using it in a real fight, you will have greater success kicking to the groin and then following up with hard punches.

Caution

If you have not practiced the funny kick before, go easy at first. It's quite stressful on the knee joint. Be kind to your knees and go easy the first few workouts. Trust me on this. I have had many students limp into Wednesday's class after going too hard with the funny kick in Monday's class. It's also wise not do it on the bag for several workouts until your knees get use to the motion.

First two weeks (Go easy)
Air: 2 sets, 10 reps — each leg, 2 times a week
After first two weeks (Pick up the pace but watch for knee pain)
3 sets, 15 reps — each leg, 2 times a week
After 3-4 weeks
Heavy bag: 2 sets, 15 reps —each leg, 2 times a week

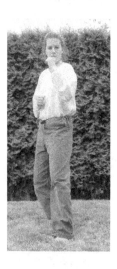
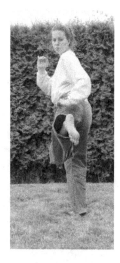

From your on-guard position, twist your upper body hard to your right as you flip out the lower portion of your led leg, striking with the little-toe side of your foot.

Groin Slap with a Hook

As if slapping your foot up into an assailant's groin isn't bad enough, the little added bonus I offer here will make his experience even more miserable. As the old saying goes: Don't pick on me if you don't want to get your groin kicked into the dirt. (Actually, I just made that up.)

The slap kick is done with either the front or rear foot; it's faster with the front and stronger with the rear. You don't have to take time to chamber your leg, since it's already bent from crouching in whatever stance you are in. When the assailant is close enough, all you have to do is straighten your leg and it snaps right up into the target. If he is out of range, close the distance by stepping up with your rear foot to the heel of your front foot, and then kick with your front foot into the target (this is the replacement step discussed on page 92, "Five Basic Ways to Step."). As you probably know, it doesn't take a lot of force against the groin to make the recipient's face turn crimson, his cheeks inflate and his eyes roll about like ping pong balls in a lotto machine.

When the top of your foot is brought straight up between the recipient's legs, anything and everything in the way gets crushed. The harder you kick, the greater the crush. But why stop with a little ol' crush? Here is an add-on you can do to really make him cry "uncle!"

Add a hook   Assume your stance, and then step up to your front foot with your rear foot and launch your front-legged slap kick with a snap of your knee. The moment your foot hits the imaginary target, point your foot upward and jerk it back as if trying to strike yourself in the chest with your knee. What happens is that after your slap kick crushes his groin against his pelvic bone, the front of your foot hooks the wounded target and then rips and tears everything in its path on its way out. I'll pause here until you stop grimacing and groaning.

Practice the following drill with a step and also without one. When stepping, move your rear foot up to your front heel and slap kick with your front foot. Think of the action of your rear foot as sort of "kicking" your lead one out of the way. As mentioned, you don't need to chamber your front leg because it's already partially bent from your stance. Just snap it up and into the target, hook it —and pull back with extreme prejudice. Make the motion fluid. Don't do it in three separate motion, such as, first, a slap kick, and then hook, and then a pull. Instead, make it one smooth motion: slaphookjerk.

In the air: 3 sets, 15 reps — both legs
Heavy bag: 3 sets, 15 reps — both legs

Scoop Kick

One karate style calls this "toe out kick," which describes exactly how the foot is formed. It was taught to me as "scoop kick," and since old habits are hard to change, I'll continue calling it that. Besides, scoop kick is also descriptive since the kick is launched in a scooping motion along the floor and up into the target where the arch of the foot makes contact.

I teach that the scoop kick should be used for the same purpose a boxer uses his jab: to harass, to set up the opponent, to measure distance and as part of a combination. It's a marvelous distraction technique, because when you pop three or four scoop kicks to a street assailant's lower leg, his brain focuses on the pain, which leaves his upper half wide open for whatever you want to do to him there.

To launch the kick, assume your fighting stance with your left leg forward. Scoot your rear foot along the floor, just grazing it, and scoop it up and into your imaginary opponent's knee. Set it down in front of you if you going to continue to advance with other blows, or return your foot to where it was initially if the scoop is all you intend to do.

The kick can also be done with the front leg, though it isn't as powerful as the rear one. You can generate a little more power by doing a replacement step (the same method you used with the slap kick), which adds forward momentum to the impact. Because it isn't as powerful as when done with the rear foot, many fighters use the front scoop simply as a way to harass and distract their opponents by keeping them busy trying to avoid the kick. It's also a good interrupter. Every time your opponent sets himself to attack, you pop a scoop against his closest leg.

The target is anywhere on the opponent's leg: front, side or back. Incidentally, the knee cap is not as easy to break as many people believe, though it's still no picnic to get hit there. If you want to use the kick as a take down when you are behind him, scoop your foot into the back of his knee, and then press forward until his kneecap makes painful contact against the asphalt. Feel free to jerk his shoulder back or pull the hair at the back of his head to hurry him down a little faster.

If you are having problems turning your foot out far enough, keep working on it until you have the necessary flexibility in your ankle. One way is to press the arch of your foot against a wall and hold it there for a minute at a time. Include this as part of your warm up and your foot will be flexible enough in no time. To keep from spraining your ankle, it's a good idea to avoid kicking the bag hard until you can turn your foot out properly.

Training Tip

In the air: 3 sets, 10 reps – both legs
Against a bag: 3 sets, 10 reps – both legs

Scoot your rear foot along the floor and into your opponent's closest knee.

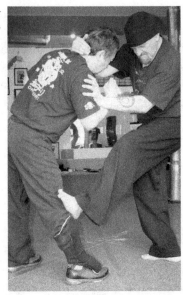

Stomp scoop: Some karate people might argue that technically this is not a scoop, but for our purposes here, it's similar enough
to include it in this section. If the situation justifies it, you can use
it to stomp an assailant's knee. Say you have knocked him against
a wall, and he is sprawled there with one leg extended before him.
Scoop your rear foot forward, and at about the half way point, draw
your knee up high and then slam the bottom of your foot down on
his bridged knee. This variation carries with it the risk of crippling
the man, so it's imperative the situation justifies that level of force.
For example, you would be justified if he was armed with a knife or
club, but him calling your mother a name is not enough reason for
you to give him a permanent limp. Trust me, lawsuits are not fun.

In the air: 3 sets, 15 reps — both legs
On the bag: 3 sets, 15 reps — both legs

Angle stomp scoop: There are two primary differences
with this version: You kick with the bottom of your foot, slightly
toward the outside edge of the little toe side. The other difference
is that your opponent is lying on the ground.

The kick begins with a high chamber. Lift your knee up to the
front of your body and position your kicking foot in front of your
groin as you angle your knee outward slightly. The kick is executed
with a powerful, angled thrust across the front of your support leg
and downward to the target, which is your opponent's head or body.
To add greater power to the kick, arch your back a little just prior
to your foot making contact. This is a wonderful technique to use
as a follow-up after a take down.

Training
Tip

Air kicks: 3 sets, 10 reps — both legs
Prone bag kicks: 3 sets, 10 reps — both legs

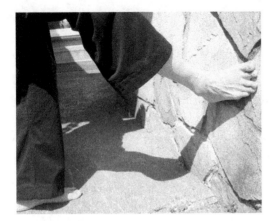

To build flexibility
in your ankle, press
the arch of your
foot against a wall,
twist your foot
outward and hold
for one minute.

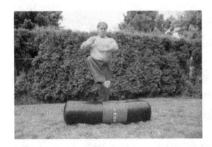

Pantomiming that you are
holding onto the arm of
someone you have dumped on
the ground, lift your foot up
near your groin. Thrust your
foot downward at an angle into
your opponent's head.

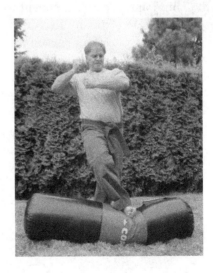

Inside-knee strike

Some Muay Thai fighters call this "inside-knee strike" while others call it "curve kick." I call it inside-knee strike since it better describes the action of your leg. The strike is used when you are literally stomach to stomach with your opponent in a clinch, an often awkward position where it's nearly impossible to deliver a front or rear knee strike with significant force.

Partners

To do it against a live opponent, snuggle up close, wrap your hands around the back of his neck and pull him into your blow. Press your forearms close together to make it difficult for him to punch you in the body. Stay light on your feet, shifting your weight back and forth as you jerk your opponent around. Come up on the ball of your left foot as you swing your bent right leg away from your opponent's side, and then forcefully swing it back into him, striking his ribs with the inside area of your knee. Striking his ribs, especially the so-called floating rib just beneath his rib cage, causes him pain and nausea. I also like to strike the outside of his hips because impact there sometimes collapses the supporting leg.

Instructor Frank Garza agrees. "The key to this particular knee is to be belly to belly and then slyly move your knee out and then into his body. Anything you hit with this technique, ribs, kidney, hip joint, gets the opponent to drop his hands, which opens him up for an elbow to the face. The only problem I can see is when you haven't yet softened up your opponent. Then when you lift your knee, he can trip your support leg and you're in for a nasty fall. But every technique has a downside when it's not setup properly. But, wow, talk about an effective technique; this is a good one."

To practice the inside knee strike by your lonesome, hug your heavy bag, a manikin or even a padded pole. Alternate striking the sides of your target with both knees, striving for stability while staying in motion on your feet. Be sure to pull the bag into the strike for added impact. If you are doing it on an immovable pole, pull with your arms anyway just to establish the habit.

3 sets, 10 reps -- both legs

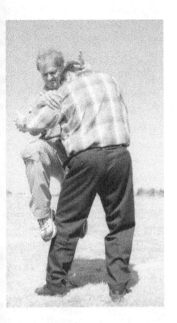 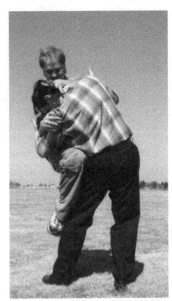

From a tight clinch, angle your right knee outward, and then slam it into your assailant's lower rib area.

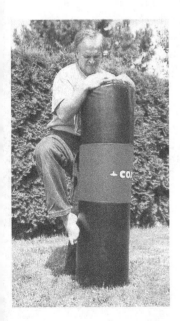 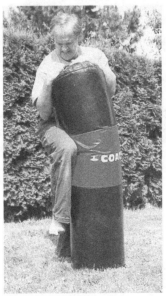

Hug your heavy bag close to your chest as you angle your knee outward and then slam it in hard. In the first photo, my knee is fairly close to the bag. You can also practice with your knee pointing all the way to the side prior to slamming the bag.

Outside Crescent Kick

While the outside crescent kick isn't as off-the-beaten path as the last four, I like it so much that I have included it here just to encourage you to work on it. An outside crescent is one where your leg arcs away from your body as opposed to an inside crescent, which arcs across the front of your body. I prefer the outside version because it's faster and it isn't as hard on the knee. Once, a high-ranking martial artist argued that it wasn't a good kick, but then he changed his mind when he had trouble holding the bag for one of my students who, at 135 pounds, can nearly shred a hand-held bag with it. There are two variations of the outside crescent: front leg and rear leg.

Front-leg outside crescent   Assume a left-leg-forward stance and face your imaginary opponent who is standing at 12 o'clock. Step up with your rear foot just behind your left and snap your left foot up with a slightly bent leg toward 2 o'clock. When it reaches whatever height you want, whip it toward your imaginary opponent, hitting the target with the outer edge, the little toe side, of your foot. Its power comes from speed, hip rotation and a slight snap of your knee. Don't tense your leg or hip muscles in an attempt to hit hard. Strive for smoothness and speed and power will come naturally.

Training Tip

Time your crescent, whether you are kicking to a high target or a low one, so that you make contact at the apex of the arc. I like to kick low with it -- kidney, groin and inside of the thigh -- so the arc isn't as pronounced as it is when kicking high. But that is okay because a low crescent still hurts. With practice, your speed, muscle development and application of proper body mechanics may make the crescent one of your favorite kicks.

Rear-leg outside crescent   Crescent kicking to the outside with the rear leg isn't as fast as with the front leg but it's more powerful and quite deceptive. Be careful that you don't hook your front ankle with your rear foot as it passes; it not only hurts like the dickens, but you look stupid when it happens (been there, done that). If you are just learning the rear crescent, try this variation taught by

Instructor Alain Burrese. Here is how he describes it.

"Assume your fighting stance face to face with the heavy bag, right leg back. Step off to the left at a 45-degree angle or so. The right leg goes straight up to 12 o'clock and then snaps to the right into the bag, connecting with the outside of the foot. Switch stances and repeat on the other side."

When you move at an angle to your opponent, he is momentarily confused as to what you are doing. His eyes follow as you step to your left, and then he sees your rear foot shoot straight up at his side, two feet away from him. Just as he starts to think, "What the --," your foot slaps into his groin.

The crescent kick with either leg will chalk up points in competition because it's impressive when snapped to the opponent's face and it makes a resounding slapping noise when whipped into his upper body. It's especially pertinent for the street because it can be delivered with very little telegraphing against vulnerable targets, such as the groin, inner thigh, outer thigh, back of knee and kidneys.

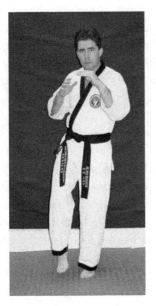

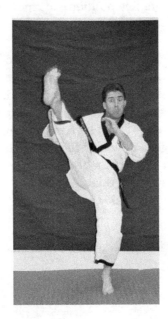

Instructor Alain Burrese steps off to the left with his lead foot and begins moving his rright foot forward and up into an outside crescent kick.

Exercises and drills for the crescent kicks

Try the following exercises to develop speed, power and flexibility for the crescent kick.

Front-leg outside crescent:
Air reps: 3 sets, 10 reps – both legs,
Heavy bag: 3 sets, 10 reps – both legs

Rear-leg outside crescents:
Air reps: 3 sets, 10 reps – both legs
Heavy bag: 3 sets, 10 reps – both legs

Supported slow motion kicks: Hold on to the back of a kitchen chair, or anything else that works, with your left leg forward. That grease spot on the wall in front of you at 12 o'clock is your opponent. Slowly lift your slightly bent left leg up toward 2 o'clock as high as you are able. Even if you never kick high, do so when you exercise your crescent to more intensely stimulate the involved muscles. When you have reached your maximum height, strain to lift your leg even higher. Yes it hurts, but move your leg slowly in an arc toward that spot on the wall. Bring your foot straight down to its beginning position and repeat. Do these slowly and eat the pain.
2 sets, 10 reps — each leg

Workout
Tip

Kick over the chair: Here is another kitchen chair exercise, one that has a built-in incentive. Face the chair in your fighting stance, step up with your rear foot and execute a slow crescent over the chair's back. I strongly suggest doing them slowly at first because if you don't kick high enough or your leg is somehow off course, you get a not-so-friendly reminder in the form of a crunched toe. Once you get the feel of distance and height, kick over the chair as fast as you want.
3 sets, 10 reps — each leg

Kick over a standing bag: Hapkido instructor Alain Burrese uses this exercise to work all the muscles involved with the crescent kick, especially the hips. You may not like to kick as high as this requires, nonetheless use it as an exercise to loosen and strengthen all the involved muscles. Use a freestanding bag or, if you don't have one, use a pile of boxes or tires. Stand in front of it with your left leg forward. Step up with your rear leg and quickly lift your front leg up the right side of the bag, swing it over the top and down the left side. Aim with the outside edge of your foot throughout the movement.

2 sets, 15 reps — each leg

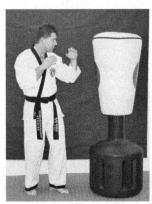

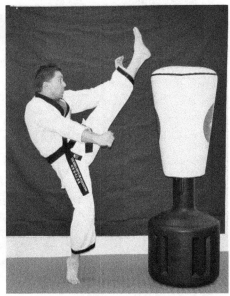

From an on-guard position, Instructor Burrese steps up to the bag using a replacement step, and then kicks up and over it.

Bungee cord: This exercise works great, feels great and hits the exact muscles involved in the crescent kick. It also makes it hard for you to walk the next day if, in your enthusiasm, you begin with too many sets and reps. Train smart and start out with one set and progress to three.

Attach the cord to your right ankle and lie on your left side. Extend your left arm along the floor for balance and cross your right leg over your left. Scoot yourself away from whatever you have the cord attached to until the cord is tight. Remember, you hit with the outer edge of your foot, so position your foot accordingly as you slowly lift your leg straight up. You can either stop there and return it to the floor, or you can go beyond the straight up position to get a little extra stretch and resistance in the rep.

1-3 sets, 15 reps — each leg

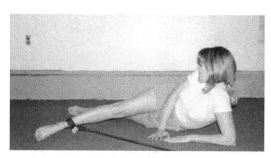

Position yourself so the cord is taught. Slowly bring your crescent kick straight up and then back to the starting position.

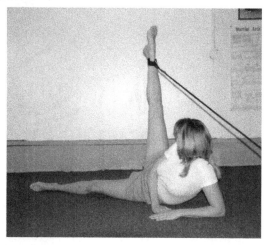

LEAD LEG KICKS

Most kicks can be done with either your lead leg or your rear leg and, as a general rule, the rear leg is more powerful, while the lead leg is quicker. Years ago, martial artists used to argue that lead-leg kicks were weak, but when champion full-contact fighter Bill Wallace and others began knocking opponents unconscious with their lead kicks, the arguments died a quick death.

As a street-oriented stylist, I emphasize that my students use mostly lead kicks in their training and aim for vulnerable targets, such as the inner and outer thigh, knee, groin, solar plexus and kidneys. My reasoning is this:

- The lead is closest to the opponent
- It's faster than the rear leg
- There is less telegraphing, which means there is less time for the opponent to defend
- There is less body leaning (at least there should be)
- It's easier to follow the kick with punches

There is nothing exotic about the following exercise; you probably do lots of lead-leg kicking now. I'm suggesting, however, that you practice the kicks with a mindset that you are in competition or in a street self-defense situation, and it's imperative that you launch your kicks with speed and accuracy. *Concentrate* on each kick to bring out your best. Such as:

Important

- Concentrate on throwing it without preparatory movement
- Concentrate on launching it as quick as a wink
- Concentrate on where you want to hit (use a manikin-type bag, or if you have a heavy bag, put pieces of tape on it to represent targets)
- Think about what you would do as a follow-up

To reiterate, don't just mindlessly throw out these lead-leg kicks. Think about each rep so that the reason behind it is imprinted in your mind.

Front kick - 2 sets, 10 reps —each side
Side kick - 2 sets, 10 reps — each side
Roundhouse kick - 2 sets, 10 reps — each side
Back kick - 2 sets, 10 reps — each side
Your favorite kick(s) other than the basic four: 2 sets, 10 reps — each side

ONE LEGGED NONSTOP KICKS

To do this exercise, lift your right leg and throw every kick in your arsenal for 60 seconds before you return your foot to the floor. Then lift your left leg and do every kick you know for 60 seconds. Continue alternating your legs for as long as you can without spewing up your last meal.

This is a tough one that works your cardiovascular system, the muscles of your legs, hips and your balance. A valuable side benefit is that you become acutely aware of the necessary body mechanics of each kick. When you do a front kick rep, followed by a hook kick, followed by a back kick, all with the same leg, you develop a greater understanding of your support foot placement and all the necessary body turning, twisting and leaning needed to perform each kick.

Perform each rep with power, speed and snap, striving for fast retractions and fast body shifts that position you for the next kick. As you get tired, strive to keep your form perfect. Fatigue is not an excuse to throw out sloppy kicks. Aim for perfection no matter how drained your energy.

3 sets, 60 seconds per leg, 30–60 kicks per minute (both legs counts as 1 set)

THE LAST LEG EXERCISE

I call this "The last leg exercise" because after you have completed it, it's the last thing you do that day. I stole it from something I read on Ultimate Fighting Champion Ken Shamrock, who uses this to develop leg strength and overall endurance. You can do it for that, too, or you can do it when you really want to trash the ol' gams. It's tough, but if done regularly, your legs and your discipline will be ironclad. Here is how it's done.

Deep, body-weight squats: 1 set, 500 reps

No, that is not a typo, you really do 500 squats. Although, Shamrock may do one giant set of them, arguably that is not as productive as breaking them into sets with a 15-30 second rest in between. No matter how you break it up, 500 reps makes for a tough workout, so you shouldn't do it more than once every two or three weeks.

You can be like Shamrock and do all of them at once, or you can split them, such as:

5 sets, 100 reps
10 sets, 50 reps
25 sets, 20 reps
50 sets, 10 reps

When Shamrock finishes his 500, he drops to the floor and burns out as many crunches as he can. He then finishes his workout by rolling over and doing three sets of push-ups, each set to failure. What an animal!

LEG CHAMBERING EXERCISES

If you can't chamber your kicks quickly and effortlessly, your kicks will never reach their full potential. The muscles that chamber your legs get lots of work anytime you practice kicking drills, reps, kata, and sparring, but they benefit even more when you do specific exercises that develop their strength, speed and flexibility. Greater strength means less effort to lift your legs into a chamber, which facilitates the speed of the action. Faster chambering means less setup time for your kick, which ultimately leads to faster delivery of your foot to the target. The more flexible you are, the higher you can chamber and therefore the higher your kick. This is important for high kickers, but flexibility is also important for fighters who favor kicking to low targets, since flexible muscles help enable you to kick with greater speed. Interesting how it all blends together, isn't it? Let's look at some exercises that improve all three areas.

Important

Building Strength in the Chamber

The following exercises build strength in your hips so you can chamber your leg with speed and kick with power.

Front kick chamber with kick   You may do this exercise holding onto a support, though your eventual goal is to do it unsupported. Chamber your right leg as high as you are able and then use your hand to lift it even higher. Hold for 10 seconds. Remove your hands and execute a medium speed front kick as high as you can. Return to the chamber and repeat the entire procedure.
1 set, 10 reps — each leg

Front kick chamber and hold   Chamber your front kick as before and use your hand to lift it even higher. This time, hold it for 30 seconds and then lower your foot to the ground without kicking. Do 10 reps, but use your hip and leg muscles on the last three to keep your chamber as high as possible with just a minimum of help from your hands.
1 set, 10 reps — each leg

Building Speed in your Chamber

Before we look at the exercises, allow me to make a little announcement here. If you are less than 30 years of age, you probably won't believe what I'm going to say, but if you are over 30, you understand exactly what I'm saying. Here is my announcement: Your joints—shoulders, elbows, hips and knees—are not going to tolerate your snapping them in the air and slamming heavy bags forever. While there are some people who can get away with it for several years without a problem, there are others who cannot.

Important

Which one are you? You don't know, and that is the problem. If you go 30 years before your joints start to rebel, you know then that you are one of the lucky ones, but if you train for only four years before you start having problems or have irreparable damage, you are not so lucky. Since you have no way of knowing which category you are in, does it not make sense to baby them from the get go?

But how can you take it easy when proficiency in the martial arts requires lots and lots of repetitions in the air and on the bag? The solution is simple: Don't do all your reps at maximum speed and power. I understand that is a concept that is hard to accept for fighters who think that every rep must be slammed out as if they are fighting for their lives. If you are one of these people, you have to change your way of thinking if you want to enjoy the fighting arts for many years.

I'm continuously searching for exercises that develop technique, power and speed but do not require pounding out bone-wearing reps. The good news is that there are plenty of them out there; the bad news is that I didn't discover them until about 10 years ago. But better late than never. I'm convinced that I'm still training because I made the switch in my thinking. I encourage you to also explore exercises and drills that are easy on your joints.

Here are eight exercises that are easy on your hip bones, but still develop the muscles necessary for a fast chamber. They are not easy, so grit your teeth and, as they say in those hanging-fern restaurants—enjoy.

—

Front knee chamber   Up against the wall! Although I uttered those four words a few hundred times during my police career, this time I'm saying them to get you in position to work on developing fast chambers. If you haven't got a wall, which is a little hard to imagine, use the back of a kitchen chair. This is an easy-on-your-joints exercise that develops flexibility and speed in the chambering portion of your front kick, and any other kick that begins similarly. It also gets you huffing and puffing, which makes for an excellent aerobic workout. If you lift weights, consider doing these between sets to keep your heart rate elevated.

Place your palms on a wall at about shoulder height and position your feet side-by-side about two feet back. Incline your body about 45 degrees toward the wall and then raise your left knee as high as you are able. Set it down and immediately raise your right one as high as you can. Think of striking yourself in the chest with your knees as you alternate as fast and as high as you can.

3 sets, 25-50 reps — each knee

Roundhouse chamber   Support yourself on a wall or chair with one hand and lean slightly to the side as you do when executing your roundhouse kick. Turn your stationary foot away from the direction you are kicking and keep it in that position as you snap up your roundhouse chamber and then lower it. Keep your stationary foot turned as you repetitiously snap your chamber up and down. You can either touch your foot to the floor each time or stop it an inch short. Push yourself to go faster and faster.

3 sets, 20 reps — each leg

Side kick chamber   Use the same format you used with the roundhouse chamber. The difference is that you lift your knee closer to your midsection (if your style chambers it differently, do this exercise anyway; it's good for you), and position the bottom or the edge of your foot toward the imaginary target. Do it for speed.

3 sets of 20 reps — each leg

Double side kick chamber   How you return your side kick is very important. When you return your kick on the same path as it went out on, you unconsciously kick correctly out to the target.

A common error beginners make, however, is to launch their side kick out and then return it by snapping their heel back toward their rear, as if they had just thrown a roundhouse kick After a few of these, their side kick begins going out to the target more like a roundhouse. To correct this, they need to stress returning the side kick on the *same* path it went out on.

Training Tip

I got this simple exercise from a taekwondo friend, and I've used it for years because it not only develops speed, but it ensures that the retraction is done properly. Chamber your leg as you normally do when side kicking, launch the kick and then retract your leg all the way back into the same tight chamber you used to launch it. You get two chambers per kick, which arguably develops your side kick twice as fast.

3 sets, 10 reps — each leg

Note: While the double side kick chamber is a good exercise and learning device, the extra time it takes to tightly chamber your leg after you have kicked might get you scored on in competition or hurt when defending yourself against a skilled fighter. Therefore, consider this only as an exercise. When applying the side kick in a tournament or the street, bring your leg back about 12 inches and then quickly set it down and continue hitting.

Experiment with half and full chambers   Many side kick experts say that chambering your knee next to your chest is sort of like stretching the rubber band all the way back on a slingshot: The rock flies fast and far (or until the neighbor's window stops it). Other fighters, however, chamber their sidekicks loosely, say half way, in the belief that the kick will reach the target faster. Opponents of half chambering agree that it's faster, but they argue that it's weaker. Using the slingshot analogy, if you pull the pouch on the slingshot back only half way, the rock will not hit the target as hard as it does when the pouch is pulled back all the way. Those who advocate the chest-hugging side kick chamber say that it may not be quite as fast as a partial chamber, but it's twice as powerful. What to believe?

Use your solo time to experiment with your kick. Chamber your side kick as tight as you can and drive your foot into your heavy bag. Do a few reps to get a good feel for the impact. Next, chamber your side kick loosely, say half of what you usually do and drive that into the bag. Do several reps and make whatever body adjustments you think will increase the impact.

I'm guessing that you will find that the tighter chamber is stronger, but did you find much of a difference in speed between the two delivery methods? I'm guessing again that you found the half chamber to be faster, but is it so much faster that you are willing to sacrifice the power? It's your call. Use your training alone time to experiment and find an answer you can live with.

Half chambers: 3 sets, 10 reps – both legs
Tight chamber: 3 sets, 10 reps – both legs

Fire hydrant roundhouses   I learned this move from my dog, although we have different objectives. Get on your hands and knees and lift your leg as high as you can into a roundhouse chamber. Push for speed and height.

3 sets, 20 reps — each leg

Begin on your hands and knees and repetitiously lift your leg into a roundhouse chamber as fast and high as you can. Lower and repeat.

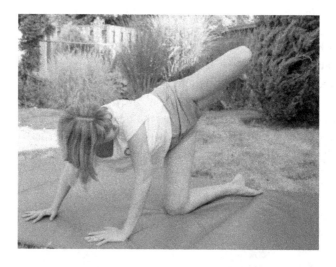

Fire hydrant side kick chambers   Because you are on your hands and knees, you can't chamber your side kick as tightly as you do when standing. No problem. The motion, though limited, will still work the fast twitch muscles.

Get on all fours and place both of your hands on the floor off to the far left to provide room for your right leg to chamber. Lift and tuck your right knee across your chest in a side kick chamber as close to your arms as you are able. Go for speed.

3 sets, 20 reps — each leg

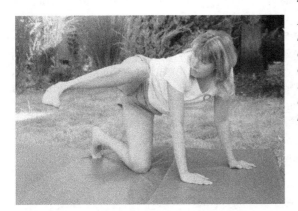

Begin on your hands and knees and, as fast as you can, lift your leg into a high sidekick chamber. Lower and repeat.

In the pool   If you have access to a pool, try any of the aforementioned chambering exercises in the water. The constant resistance works your muscles so hard that you don't need to do as many reps as when you do them on dry land. Work the front, round and side chambers.

1-2 sets, 10 reps – both legs for each exercise

If you do all of these exercises in the same workout, you will walk oddly the next day. So that you don't overtrain or strain something, especially in that area "where the sun don't shine," choose only one exercise for the front kick, one for the roundhouse and one for the side kick. Exercise your chambers twice a week, changing the exercises every third workout.

Developing a Flexible Chamber

___Knee pulls dramatically increase flexibility in your hips and abductors so that the chamber portion of your kick as well the kick itself will have a greater range and ease of motion. As mentioned earlier, even if you don't normally kick high, a flexible chamber will help you kick fast to low targets. Here are a few exercises that involve pulling your leg into a higher chamber. If you already do these, you know they are goodies. If you have never done them, you will soon be saying, "Oh man, I wish I had done these a long time ago."

Roundhouse chamber   Rest your left hand against a wall and pivot your support leg and foot as far as you usually do, anywhere from 90 to 170 degrees away from the invisible target, and lean your upper body away as far as you normally do when you kick. Lift your right, roundhouse chamber high and tight with your foot as close to your butt as possible. Take your right hand and grab the knee of your chambered leg and pull it up even higher. Keep pulling until your leg is at its maximum height, and then hold.
2 sets, 10 reps, 10–30 seconds – both legs

Rest one hand on a wall and lift your leg into a high roundhouse chamber. Use your hand to pull you leg even higher.

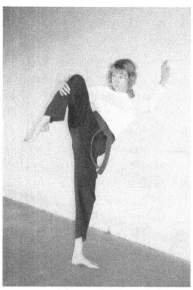

Side kick chambers   It's a little more awkward to pull up your side kick than it is the roundhouse chamber, but you can do it. Tuck your knee against your chest and pull your shin as high as you can and hold. It's that "hold" that hurts, but grit your teeth and do it anyway. If it helps, shout out, "I can eat the pain!" You will be glad you did when you see the results.

2 sets, 10 reps, 10-30 seconds — each leg

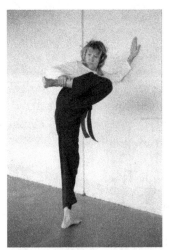

Support yourself against a wall and lift your leg into a high sidekick chamber with your knee tucked as close to your chest as possible. Use your hand to pull your leg even higher.

Front kick chamber   Lean back against a wall and pull your right knee toward your chest as high as you are able. Use one or both of your hands to lift it even higher.

2 sets, 10 reps, 10-30 seconds -- both legs

STOP SWATTING MOSQUITOES

A common error among beginners, and occasionally among advanced students who have picked up this bad habit, is something I call "swatting mosquitoes." I'm talking about fighters who wave their arms about as they kick. It might be one arm up over the head and the other out to the side, or both arms may flail about in any number of ways. If this is you, you need to correct the problem immediately; it's important to be in control of every part of your body because every part of your body is involved in the kick.

Sometimes it might seem that spreading your arms helps your kick, but it doesn't and may even throw you off balance. It also makes it hard for you to act offensively and defensively. If that kick gets blocked and your opponent scoots in fast with a counter punch to your chest, you are going to have a hard time blocking when your arms are waving all over the place. And just try to follow your kick with a fast punch when one of your arms is pointing high right and the other is pointing low left.

Grab your Shirt

Try holding onto the front of your T-shirt or uniform jacket when you practice your kicking reps. This places your hands close to where they should be, but more importantly, it draws your attention to what they are doing. I've seen students eliminate their arm waving in one class using this gimmick.

The Wooden Dowel and Rope Trick

Here are two other methods to correct swatting mosquitoes suggested by Instructor David Giles that you can experiment with when training alone.

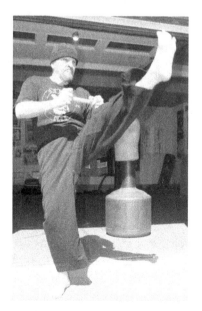

"This is really quite simple," Giles says. "While working kicks on the heavy bag, raise your hands to your on-guard position. In order to ensure that they stay there, hold a length of wooden doweling (dowels are cheap, so you can custom-cut them) between your palms and keep it there throughout your kicking routine. If you try to balance yourself by flinging your arms out, you will drop the dowel.

It's a beginner's level drill, but it helped me get rid of the problem. It definitely helps one be aware of where his hands are.

"If you have problems with pressing your hands together when you kick, substitute a length of rope or a belt for the dowel. With this, your objective is to keep it taut throughout the drill. If it goes slack, you know you are bringing your hands together."

There are kicks that involve whipping your arms to help accelerate the action, but you need to have control of your arms before you can use them. Gimmicks such as holding your shirt, holding a wooden dowel or length of rope will help you keep your hands where you can use them.

To keep from pressing your hands together, hold a rope or pants belt in your hands.

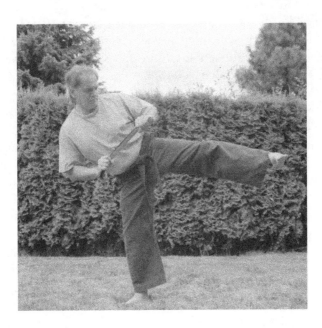

EXERCISES TO DEVELOP SPEED, POWER, ENDURANCE & ACCURACY

Here are a few exercises that develop speed, power, dexterity and endurance in all of the kicks we have discussed in this section. Work hard and consistently on these and you will enjoy tremendous progress that will inspire you to keep training even harder.

8, 2-minute Rounds, 4 Kicks

This tough exercise uses the four basic kicks to improve your sparring and definitely gets your heart racing and your lungs burning. It will sharpen your front, round, side and back kicks, which in turn will improve all of your others. Of course, you can replace one or more of the basics with any other kick you want to improve.

This exercise is also the perfect device to strengthen your discipline because once you are into it, you want it to be over. You will have to draw upon your fortitude to keep at it since "keeping at it" is what the martial arts are all about. Yes, it's a toughie, but it's also a goodie. Here is how it works.

Front kick only   Assuming you are warmed up and raring to go, begin with the front kick. Set the kitchen egg timer for two minutes and begin moving around as if sparring an opponent. Attack your invisible friend only with front kicks and when he attacks you with his imaginary punches and kicks, block them, and counter only with front kicks.

You have 120 seconds in every 2-minute round, so you need to push yourself to front kick at least 100 times during each round. Be sure to include shuffling, bobbing, weaving and blocking, but not so much that you can't get in your 100, which is the purpose of the drill. At the end of 2 minutes, rest for 1 minute, and then do another 2-minute round of front kicks, again pushing to do at least 100 of them.

Roundhouse kick only____ After your second all-too-short 1-minute rest, crank up the timer for another round. This time do roundhouse kicks, including blocking and as much bobbing, weaving and shuffling as you can manage while still getting in at least 100 reps. Rest 1 minute and then do another 2 minutes of roundhouse kicks.

Side kicks only____ This time it's side kicks for 2, 2-minute rounds, banging out at least 100, with as much blocking, bobbing, weaving and shuffling as you can get in.

Back kicks only   Back kicks only for 2, 2-minute rounds. Again, strive for a minimum of 100.

Your objective is to kick hard and fast. Over the weeks, increase the number of kicks that you do within the 2-minute rounds, but monitor yourself to ensure you are executing them flawlessly. The drill is ineffective if your kicks are executed improperly.

Important

You will no doubt feel like warmed over roadkill at the end of the eight rounds, and for good reason: you just threw at least 800 hard kicks. Your cardio will improve in time and you may find yourself wanting to add a third round. This is fine, but add just one round at a time. For example, the first week you want to increase your output, add one round for the front kick. The next week, add one for the roundhouses, and so on. Progress wisely and you will develop a strong cardiovascular system without killing yourself. Remember, your primary objective is to develop strong, fast and *perfect* techniques.

Here is the drill in a package:

Round 1: front kick	*minimum 100 reps*	*2 minutes, rest 1 minute*
Round 2: front kick	*minimum 100 reps*	*2 minutes, rest 1 minute*
Round 3: roundhouse	*minimum 100 reps*	*2 minutes, rest 1 minute*
Round 4: roundhouse	*minimum 100 reps*	*2 minutes, rest* 1 minute
Round 5: side kick	*minimum 100 reps*	*2 minutes, rest 1 minute*
Round 6: side kick	*minimum 100 reps*	*2 minutes, rest 1 minute*
Round 7 back kick	*minimum 100 reps*	*2 minutes, rest 1 minute*
Round 8 back kick	*minimum 100 reps*	*2 minutes, collapse*

How to prioritize It's a good idea to prioritize the order of your two-minute rounds by beginning with whatever kick needs the most work. If your side kick is not as polished as it should be, begin the exercise with it since you have your most energy during the beginning of the drill. If your back kick is your best one, do it last. This doesn't mean you take it easy with the back kick, but since it needs the least work, do it when you have the least energy.

I have illustrated the 8, 2-Minute Rounds, 4 Kicks Drill using the basic kicks because they work all the muscles used in most other leg techniques. But it's not mandatory that you do only the four basic ones. As mentioned, you are free to insert whatever ones you want to sharpen. You might want to include two basic kicks and two that you like that are more esoteric. Of course, you can make all four kicks esoteric ones. That is the beauty of training alone; it's your drill, do it the way that benefits you the most.

Kicking Balloons

Admittedly, it's not easy to buy a bag of birthday party balloons when you are a big, tough, karate guy, but swallow your pride and do it anyway because the following exercise is a good one. If it helps, buy all menacing-looking black ones and avoid the pretty yellows, pinks and those with clowns on them. But if you hate clowns . . .

The exercise is to simply kick a balloon all about. While you may be tempted to inflate several and create a fun and festive atmosphere in your training area, fight the urge and inflate just one. Toss it in the air and kick it as long as you are able without letting it touch the floor. It's not about kicking hard, but accurately and at the right angle to keep it airborne. Use only one kick to keep it going, or use two of your favorites. Heck, you may want to use your entire repertoire of kicks to keep it bouncing about the airstreams.

To make it more interesting and street realistic, clutter your training area with hand-held pads, gloves, training bags and sticks. The idea is to keep the balloon afloat while not tripping over things on the floor and toppling out an open window. It's a challenge because you have to keep your eyes on the floating balloon while being careful of what is lying at your feet. The same situation often exists on the street or in a crowded establishment.

3 sets, 5-minutes increments

Pole Climbing

I talked about doing a variation of this exercise with a partner in *Fighter's Fact Book*, but you can also do it alone using a tree or pole. Since this requires that you keep your leg up for an extended time, it's a great exercise for developing hip power, and since you are kicking to different heights, you also develop muscle control so you can kick with greater accuracy. Here is how you do it.

To designate targets at various heights, use chalk, ink or those colored stick-ons, and put the lowest one about 12 inches from the floor, then another three feet up from the floor, four feet, five feet and one at the six-foot mark. If you want more targets, feel free to add them, but you might want to wait until you have experienced the exercise a couple times. Make sure you are thoroughly stretched and then position yourself before the pole in your fighting stance.

Execute a front kick at the lowest mark, retract quickly to your chambered position and then kick at the next highest target. Retract your foot and then kick at the next highest mark and continue in this fashion, never touching the ground, until you have kicked at the highest mark you can. Since you don't get the luxury of setting your kicking foot back on the floor between kicks, you may hear your hips cry out for mercy. But don't give it to them.

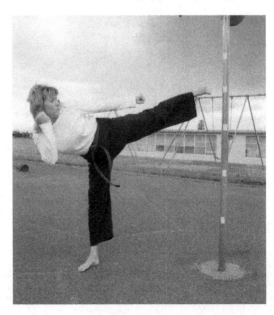

One time up the pole, no matter how many targets you kick at, counts as one rep. So if you kick at five targets, one rep is actually five kicks. Five reps, equals 25 kicks. Begin with 5 reps per kick with each leg.

Here is a sample workout

that you should try the first time you do this exercise. You choose the number of targets, though there should be at least five. If it's too hard, reduce the reps to two. If it's too easy, increase the reps to four or five and increase the number of targets.

Front kick: 5 reps – each leg
Roundhouse kick: 5 reps – each leg
Side kick: 5 reps – each leg
Straight back kick (no turn): 5 reps – each leg

Here are some ways to modify the exercise. Feel free to create more of your own.

- Increase the number of targets
- Kick on the way up the pole and on the way down on each rep
- Kick twice at each target
- Execute a different kick at each target
- Do all 5 reps of each kick in the sample workout with out returning your foot to the floor.

Workout
Tip

Double Kicks

Here is another drill to work your basics, especially your hip muscles. As the name implies, you do two kicks per count.

It's arguable whether double kicks, with the same leg, are valid for street fighting. I think it depends on the kicker. Some fighters are strong, fast, and tricky enough to be successful at it, while others only think they are. Many of the latter are those I call the flippy-dippy kickers, people who throw out tapping-type kicks that look impressive against an opponent but would have a street thug laughing uproariously before he dumped the kicker on his skull. Unfortunately, many of these double kickers have never gone near a heavy bag but have gotten their confidence from no-contact sparring and air kicking. Confidence based on false assumptions is a bad thing and can be dangerous to your health.

What is not an assumption is that you can develop powerful kicks using double kicks as a training exercise. Practice them one or two times a week by yourself, and watch the speed and power of your double kicks increase as well as the speed and power of your singular ones. Whether double kicks are applicable for self-defense is a determination you make after you have practiced the exercises for a few months and after critiquing yourself on a heavy bag and/ or on an opponent wearing protective gear.

There are two kinds of double kicks: two kicks delivered with the same leg, and one kick delivered with each leg. Let's begin by examining a few kicking exercises that will improve your ability to kick twice with the same leg.

Double kicks with same leg   Keep in mind that both kicks can be the same, such as two roundhouse kicks, or each kick can be different, such as a front kick followed by a roundhouse. The two kicks can be to different targets or to the same one.

No return to the floor: This is probably the hardest for most people because it requires a great deal of hip and leg strength. With the roundhouse kick, for example, you chamber your right leg, pop out a kick, snap it back to the chambered position, and then throw another roundhouse kick. Most people can throw a good first kick, but the second one is often slower and weaker, sometimes to the point of being feeble. This is especially true if the first roundhouse comes from the back leg, which allows for a lot of momentum. The second kick, however, doesn't have any momentum going for it, so it gets its power from only the hinge action of the knee, the contraction of the thigh muscles and body torque. While that second kick cannot be as powerful as the first, your training objective is to make it the best it can be.

Important

By working lots of repetitions, you greatly increase the focus, balance, power and speed of both kicks, especially the second one. Work hard to deliver that second kick as fast as you can, so that speed will help make up for the lack of momentum and body weight behind it.

3 sets, 10 reps – both legs

Floor bounce: Technically, this isn't a bounce, but thinking of it as such helps you generate additional power and speed in that second kick. Do it this way with your side kick: chamber it, thrust it out, snap it back, drop it to the floor, bounce it right back up into the chambered position and thrust out another side kick. On the bounce, allow just the ball of your foot to strike the floor and then use a powerful thrust of your toes to launch your leg back up into the chamber.

You can generate tremendous power with your second kick using the floor bounce. If you step forward with some kind of footwork, your first kick will be the strongest because of the momentum. But if you stand in place and launch double sidekicks, you will probably find that your bounced kick is stronger.

Most kicks can be bounced, although you might find a few that feel weak or a little odd.

3 sets, 10 reps – both legs

Fake with first kick: Fighters who are good at this have a fairly easy time of scoring, at least the first time they do it to their opponent. It's usually harder the second time to score since the element of surprise is gone. The classic move, which has worked in tournaments for years, is to fake first to the groin with a front kick and then roll the leg into a roundhouse to a higher target. The more flexible you are, and the looser your joints, the easier you can execute the move and fool your opponent.

Your objective is to work this combination until your fake kick and real kick look as if you have joints made of rubber. The easier the combination is for you to do, the great the chance you will distract your opponent and score to the target.

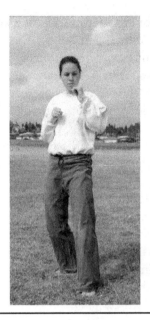 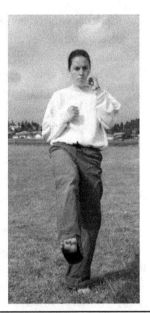

This is a classic fake seen frequently in tournaments. From the on-guard position, start to launch a front kick, Then, quick as a wink, roll your hip and roundhouse kick.

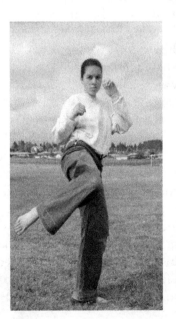 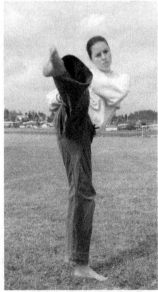

Double kicks with different legs   Throwing one kick with each leg allows you to use momentum and hip rotation for both kicks, a feature you generally don't get when throwing two kicks with the same leg. This provides you with greater power and, in some cases, greater reach. Additionally, the return of the first kick, when done with speed, will enhance the speed of the second kick, just as snapping back your arm increases the speed of your punching arm.

Important

It's important, especially in the street where fights begin and end in a matter of seconds, that your double kick is executed as efficiently as possible. To achieve this, take the time when training alone to analyze your kicks to see where you can trim the fat. Sometimes it's as simple as turning your stationary foot another two inches to allow for a more powerful second kick, or it might be a matter of rotating your hips more or less to speed up a combination. Class time is often too busy to experiment with these subtleties; that is what makes training alone so valuable.

3 sets, 10 reps – both legs for each combination

For many of my belt tests, I have students demonstrate double kicks that they have selected. This forces them to find combinations that they like and then train hard on them so they are ready to be analyzed by little ol' mean me. Because they are nervous about their pending belt test, they are going to train intensely, making a combination they like and already do well, even better. The end result is that they are going to have four or five double kicks that are top notch and serve them well in a fight.

Training alone allows you to be analytical and create combinations that suit your circumstances. Your hip structure, leg flexibility and other physical qualities are going to determine at which kicks, in this case double kicks, you excel. For example, if you have tight hips and you have done everything in the book to loosen them, but still they are tight, your roundhouse kick to the middle and side kick to the knee is going to be more effective than trying to do a roundhouse kick to the chest followed by an overhead axe kick.

Perhaps it's an injury that determines your choice of kicks. As a result of an old injury to his right knee, Bill Wallace used his left kick most of the time to defeat anyone foolish enough to take him on in the ring. I have an old hamstring injury that prevents me from kicking head high with my right leg. So my double kicks involve a relatively low right leg kick and a higher left kick.

Bad combinations   You can combine any two kicks you choose and call it a double kick. Your objective, however, is to combine kicks that flow together well, that is, kicks that have a smooth and efficient transition between them. Here is an example of a bad one: You execute a right roundhouse kick and return it to the floor in front of you. You step forward with that same foot and turn clockwise twice before you stop and execute a left, outside crescent kick. Awkward? You betcha. Efficient? Not even a little. Are there better combinations? Almost anything else.

Never lose sight of the fact that you are training to survive a real fight or to have viable techniques for competition. Choose whatever kicks you want to combine, just be sure they can be executed with the following elements.

Speed: If your transitions are coordinated and efficient, the combination will have natural speed. All you have to do then is drill on the double kick combination to build on it.

Agility: This refers to your ability to change direction and change targets quickly without wasted movement. For example, you throw a left roundhouse kick to your opponent's chest and intend to follow with a right front kick to his groin, but he blocks the roundhouse and moves three feet to the right of where he was standing. If you are agile, you can quickly adjust your body and still tag him with the front kick.

Hips and waist: This is an often neglected detail in the execution of techniques, whether you are throwing a simple punch or a double kick. Use the mirror to ensure that your hips and waist are involved in both kicks.

Timing: This is your ability to hit your opponent at the right moment. It's difficult to practice when training alone, but when all the other elements are in place as a result of good solo workouts, good timing will come quickly when you are with a training partner.

Coordination: Your coordination is there for you when all the elements of your combination have been honed and are working well together.

Efficiency: I've used the word efficiency several times because efficiency is critical to your success when throwing double kicks or, for that matter, executing any other technique. As you work your techniques, ask yourself this: Why did I just drop my arm? Why did I take that half step? Why did I lean this way? If you don't have an answer to the questions, you can probably eliminate the action. There is efficiency of movement when you trim off all that is unnecessary.

Important

3

FOOTWORK

Do you know a fighter who has great punches and kicks but can't score with them? By any chance is that fighter you? Poor footwork is common in the martial arts because footwork isn't as fun to work on as punching and kicking. Nonetheless, good footwork—meaning footwork that is fast, explosive and elusive—is vital to your success in competition and self-defense, because if you can't get your punches and kicks to the target, you are going to be a punching bag for your opponent. Incentive doesn't get much greater than that.

Admittedly, that butt-two-inches-from-the-floor horse stance looks cool and helps win kata competition, but it will get you seriously trounced in the street and, in competition, it will enable your tournament opponent to rack up points in a quick hurry. I'm not saying anything terribly profound here. When full-contact karate fighters discovered years ago that deep stances were ineffective and downright dangerous when the blows raining on them were real, they quickly converted to a stance similar to the classic boxer's. Though it's not as cool looking as the deep horse, they found that the upright position allowed them to move easily and quickly, offensively and defensively, in all directions.

Let's take a look at this stance and see why it works so well for karate.

THE BASIC BOXER STANCE

At the risk of offending boxers who may find my description too simplistic, and at the risk of boring you if you have been using the boxer's stance for a long time, allow me to give a short explanation of the stance so that we are using the same starting point for the footwork exercises that follow. The following describes a left-leg-forward fighting stance.

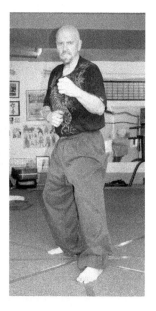

Your feet are shoulder-width apart, give or take a few inches. The 40-inch foot spread of the classic horse stance is out, while 12 to 14 inches is about as minimum as you should go. If your feet are too narrow, you have less stability. Your upper body is angled 1/4 turn from the front, making you a smaller target and allowing for maximum hip rotation when executing your techniques. When you throw a technique, your weight is usually evenly distributed, with your left foot flat on the floor and your right heel off the floor. As a rule, your lead foot points between your opponent's feet.

Changing Direction

Here is the most common and logical way to change direction when your left leg is forward (reverse the description if you fight with your right leg forward): When moving backwards or to the right, move your right foot first. When moving forward or to the left, your left foot moves first. Avoid crossing your feet so that you maintain your balance at all times. Yes, there are times when you can move the other foot first or cross your feet, but only when you are out of range of your opponent's balance-destroying charge.

Stay Moving

The continuous movement of your feet, whether making small steps or large ones, helps to camouflage your attack. Movement (your attack) from motion (movement of your body and feet) is harder for an opponent to detect than is movement from a static position. If you are out of shape aerobically (shame on you) or you are a large person and the constant motion burns up your energy, move only your upper body and keep your feet motionless. Do this by making quick bobbing and weaving motions with your upper body and jerky motions with your arms.

Training Tip

5 WAYS TO STEP

I consider the following methods of stepping to be basic because all other ways of stepping are variations of these. These are not fancy or exotic, nor should they be. I teach a street style, so we keep things simple without any bells or whistles. If you want to have fun with fancier ways of stepping, go ahead, but keep them in your kata or use them for demonstrations. Street assailants only laugh at them while they pound you into the asphalt. Here are the basic five.

Lead Lunge

This is a meat-and-potatoes step used by most fighting systems. It's a quick way to cover distances from two inches to three feet, while delivering one or more techniques. Begin by standing in your fighting stance with your left leg in front. Thrust your front foot forward so that it skims the floor while driving off the ball of your rear foot. Never lift your front foot all the way off the ground as you step because a savvy opponent can easily knock you off balance. To ensure a relatively slip-proof landing, your lead foot should land heel first, followed by the front portion of the foot, the same as when you take a normal step.

Most of the time, your rear foot moves forward just after your lead foot lands. When you lunge only to advance forward, as opposed to lunging to launch a technique, your rear foot should advance just far enough until both feet are a little wider than your shoulders. But if you are lunging to punch, your rear foot doesn't have to advance at all, though it should rotate so that it's pushing off the ball to add power to your blow.

Push for speed   To put speed into your lunge, you need to make a conscious effort to move faster and faster. It's easy for a fighter not to progress in his stepping speed because he is more conscious of his punching and kicking speed than the speed of his footwork. If you have slipped into this habit, try working your lunge without punching or kicking. Position yourself in front of your mirror and lunge forward. Move back and lunge again, each time pushing for more speed. It's easy to tense up when you push yourself, so be cognizant that you are in a state of relaxed readiness each time you explode forward.

Workout Tip

3 sets, 10 reps – each side

Replacement Step

This goes by different names but I've always used "replacement step" because it describes exactly the action of your feet. Say you are in your fighting stance with your left foot forward. To advance, move your rear foot up to the heel of your lead foot and then move your lead foot forward into another left-leg-forward fighting stance; think of kicking your lead foot forward. When attacking with hand techniques, take the same step, but move your front foot into a lead-leg-forward stance. Throughout the movement, be sure to keep your head at the same level to take advantage of the power generated by your forward momentum.

One step, 4 punches   Here is a way to fire off four techniques when doing the replacement step, a good combination to use against a "rabbit," a fighter who scrambles backwards every time you attack.

1. From your fighting stance, throw a punch with either hand but without stepping forward. This is a fake, a technique to see how your opponent reacts.
2. Move your rear foot up behind your lead. As your rear foot replaces your lead foot, fire off another hand technique.
3. As your front foot settles into forward stance, attack with two fast punches.

With repetitious practice, you will be able to execute the replacement step and punches with tremendous speed and power. To confuse and overwhelm your opponent even more, throw one blow to a high target, the next to a low one, and the next two to the middle. In step Number 2, you can replace the punch with a lead-leg kick.

No matter how proficient you become combining techniques with the replacement step, always practice a few reps of the step without punching and kicking. Be sure to keep your arms up in your on-guard position throughout the step. Push yourself to move faster and faster, all the while maintaining proper form and good balance.

Training Tip

Stepping without punching or kicking: 3 sets, 10 reps — each side
Stepping with punches and kicks: 3 sets, 10 reps — each side, each combination

Crossover Step

I stole this step from a Chuck Norris seminar I attended many years ago. I was impressed with how smoothly he executed it and how he kept his opponent so busy blocking that he was unable to counter. Although this step isn't as fast as the others we have examined, its power potential is incredible because of the forward momentum that is generated by the long step. Its lack of speed (it's still pretty darn fast) can be camouflaged by keeping your opponent busy blocking your rain storm of punches and kicks as you step over.

Get into your fighting stance with your right leg forward. To move from a right-leg-forward fighting stance to a left-leg-forward fighting stance, simply move your left foot forward until it's in the stance. If you are advancing to attack, move your left, rear foot past your lead foot until it settles into a left-leg-forward stance. The crossover step advances you the same distance as does the replacement step, but as mentioned, it has greater power.

Try this power test   Face a hanging bag with your left leg forward. Execute the crossover step as fast as you are able and, just a millisecond before your right foot settles into a right-foot-forward fighting stance, snap out a right backfist into the bag. Repeat until you can do it smoothly and with speed. Now compare that impact with a backfist thrown using a lead-leg lunge and one thrown using the replacement step. There is a big difference, isn't there? The crossover backfist is much stronger because of the tremendous forward energy accompanying your blow. Of course you would never throw a single technique with the crossover step because it would leave you open too long, making it easy for your opponent to hit you first. Instead, use a combination of blows. Here are two of many.

Combination 1: Begin with your left leg forward and throw a lead jab to feel out your imaginary opponent. As you retract your jab, move your right leg forward. As your right foot passes your lead, pop out a right backfist and then, as your foot settles into a right, forward stance, drive in two, hard punches.

Combination 2: This time pop out a left backfist to feel out your imaginary opponent. As it retracts, drive forward a front kick with your rear leg. A fraction of a second before your kicking foot sets down into forward stance, snap out a right backfist and follow with a left reverse punch.

Practice repetitiously until your crossover step and whatever hand techniques you do are smooth and fast. As with the replacement step combinations, hit targets at different levels, groin, face, midsection and face again. The idea is to confuse your opponent with blows to various heights. That, combined with your charging momentum, and your opponent is left whimpering and traumatized. Okay, I'm overstating it. But for sure he is not going to like it.

Crossover step without punches/kicks: 3 sets, 10 reps – both sides
Crossover step with punches and kicks: 3 sets, 10 reps – both sides

---

Here is a four-count hand combination using the crossover step. From your on-guard position, launch a reverse punch and then step forward, executing a second punch as your rear foot passes your lead. Snap out a backfist as your foot continues traveling forward and then a reverse punch just as your foot settles into forward stance.

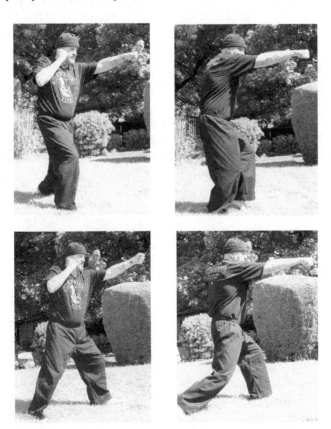

Hopping Step

You can easily cover 24-30 inches by lifting your lead leg and hopping forward on your rear foot. What you do when you get there depends on the situation. You might hop in to jam your opponent with your lead shin and then follow with a punch, or you can hop forward and kick with your lead foot. Don't kick *as* you hop because that would be a jumping kick. Instead, fire off your lead kick just as your rear foot lands.

Hopping without punches and kicks: 3 sets, 10 reps – both sides
Hopping with punches or kicks: 3 sets, 10 reps – both sides

Slide Step

The slide step is a simple way to move a few inches closer to your opponent. It's similar to the lunge, but its purpose is different. Taekwondo fighters like to use it as a way to advance before launching a lead-leg kick, but you can use it with hand techniques, too. The slide step can be used to close the distance before you punch or kick, or before you do other footwork, such as any of the stepping methods just discussed. Here are some examples:

Slide to kick   Assume your fighting stance with your left leg in front. Slide your left foot forward about 12 inches and lean your upper body forward just enough to shift your weight and advance your rear foot about half way to your lead. As soon as your rear foot lands, fire off your lead foot with whatever kick you choose.

3 sets, 10 reps - both legs

Slide to punch   From the same fighting stance, slide your left foot forward and punch. The difference between this and the lead-leg lunge is that the forward momentum of the lunge makes up part of the punch's power. With the slide, you simply close the gap and then punch. You can even pause for a second between the end of the step and your punch.

3 sets, 10 reps – both sides

Slide and step   Whatever distance you advance with the lunge, replacement, crossover and hop, you can add another 12 inches by preceding them with the slide step. One way is to move your hands about as you sneakily advance with the slide, and then explode forward with one of the steps we have talked about and with whatever punches and kicks you want.

3 sets, 10 reps – both sides

Keep your Head Level

No matter what stepping method you use to drive your punch or kick, keep your head at the same height from the takeoff point to the point of impact. When your head is maintained at a constant level, you maximize your momentum, which relies on a straight line from point A, where you begin your attack, to point B, where your hapless opponent is standing. The line is broken when that line has a bump where you raised your head and body. You may still hit him hard, but not as hard as you would have if you had kept your head level.

Important

WORKING THE ASTERISK

This is an inexpensive training device that is one of the most valuable you will own. It consists of four, five-foot strips of tape (duct tape is especially sticky and wear resistant). Tape the first two strips on the floor so they form a large plus sign, and then add the other two strips so that you now have an asterisk symbol (*), that funny-looking thing above the number 8 on your keyboard. You now have sort of a clock that has lines pointing horizontally, vertically and diagonally over its face.

When you stand in the clock's center and look forward, the line directly to your front points to 12 o'clock. The line to your rear points to 6 o'clock, straight to your right is 3 o'clock and straight to your left is 9 o'clock. Your invisible opponent is always positioned at 12. The purpose of the tape configuration is to help you "work the clock" with your footwork. Try these exercises and, as always, feel free to expand on them.

Jab and Lunge

Assume your fighting stance at the center of the clock. Jab toward 12 o'clock with your lead hand and follow a fraction of a second later with a forward lunge of your lead leg. Your lead foot should land at 12 at the same time your fist hits the imaginary opponent. You rear foot steps up to the center of the clock and you resume your on-guard position.

Lunge Back and Block

Assume your fighting stance at the center of the clock and imagine your opponent snapping a punch at your face. Simultaneously, lean away from the blow, swat it aside with your hand and lunge back with your rear foot toward 6 o'clock. Scoot your lead foot back and assume your fighting stance.

Side Step and Kick

Assume a left-leg-forward fighting stance. Step to the right toward 3 o'clock with your right leg and then launch a left roundhouse kick toward 12 o'clock.

Step Back and Punch

Assume a left-leg-forward fighting stance. As if evading an attack, move your right rear leg at an angle back to 5 o'clock, followed by a slight drag in the same direction with your left foot. When your invisible opponent starts to follow you, stop and surprise him with a hard, lunging reverse punch.

Side Step, Kick and Kick

Assume a left-leg-forward fighting stance. Step left with your left foot to 9 o'clock and snap a right side kick to 12 o'clock. Withdraw the kick, set it down next to your left, pivot and execute a left turning back kick toward 12. Set it down and resume your fighting stance.

Side Step, Block and Knee

Assume a left-leg-forward fighting stance. Step to 9 o'clock with your left leg as you backhand block your opponent's punch with your right hand. Slip your blocking hand around his head and pull it down as you slam your right knee into his middle or face.

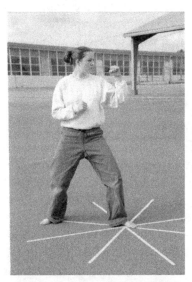

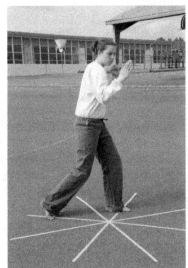

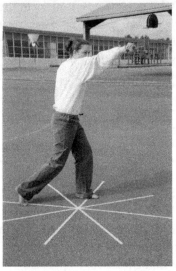

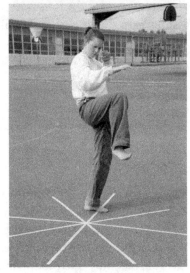

There are many combinations that you can create working the clock. It's fun, creative and it keeps your form sharp and your techniques accurate. It also develops grace under fire, so to speak. The more you practice all variations of stepping, while attacking, blocking and returning solid counters, the more likely you will do so successfully against an aggressive fighter bombarding you with punches and kicks.

Work the clock as often as you can when training alone, especially when you have found a new combination you like. Experiment with a variety of stepping patterns, and do enough repetitions with each one until you achieve smoothness. Work hard on your footwork and it will be there for you when the heat is on.

SQUAT FOR FASTER FOOTWORK

Let's finish this section on footwork with a non-martial arts exercise, but one that will develop tremendous leg power to benefit your kicks and your ability to move with explosive speed in any direction. In "The Last Leg Exercise," page 52, we discussed Ken Shamrock's weightless, high-repetition squat routine. Now let's look at two squatting exercises that use resistance.

The basic squat movement targets more muscle groups than probably any other exercise. It builds strength in the front of the thighs to generate power in all of your kicks, strong hamstrings for fast retractions and strong butt muscles to launch your kicks to the target with power and speed. Since you are exercising the largest muscles in your body, squats stimulate your heart and lungs and will have you breathing as if you have just run a couple of blocks.

Yeah, but what about my knees? you ask. The newest word from fitness experts is that squats are not bad for your knees if you do them correctly. In fact, correctly performed squats actually improve their health by strengthening them.

Machine Squats

Yeah, but what about my back? you ask. Yes, squats with a barbell can be a problem, but machines are good alternatives. Discuss your back problem with a qualified person at your gym to see which squat machines he recommends. One called the Smith is often recommended for people with bad backs.

Caution

Dumbbell Squats

If you don't go to a gym, but own dumbbells, you are in business. Grab two, position your feet about shoulder-width apart and stand straight as an arrow. Look forward, hold your chest up and shift your weight to your heels. Lower yourself as if you were going to sit down and keep going until your thighs are parallel with the ground. Pause for half a second and then push yourself up to the standing position. At the top, tilt your pelvis forward slightly to fully contract every muscle in your body.

It's been said that a fighter is only as good as his legs, and it's true. The stronger and faster your kicks, the harder they hit when they get to the target. Squats will not only give you speed and power for killer kicks, but also an improved ability to move forwards, backwards, sideways and diagonally, and do so like an exploding bomb. Your thrust will be stronger, as will your balance when executing techniques while moving. You will especially see a difference in your ability to move fast from an immobile position, such as standing casually or leaning against a wall. That ability could save your bacon in a self-defense situation.

Here is the good news. Since you probably get plenty of leg exercise during the week in your karate training, there is no advantage to doing squats more than once a week. Work them hard when you have at least one day off before your next karate training. Two days of rest is even better. Try squats for three months (12-15 workouts), and be prepared to see a big difference in how you move.

Squats: 4-5 sets, 10-15 reps – once a week

Workout
Tip

4

HANDS, ELBOWS AND FOREARMS

I hate these kinds of questions: "Which fighting style is best?" and "Which is better to use in a fight, feet or fists?" There is no blanket answer to these questions because there are just too many variables involved. Nonetheless, we can make some observations. For example, while some taekwondo tournaments are won mostly with kicking techniques, most open tournaments are won with hand strikes. Out in the mean streets, most veteran street brawlers agree that real fights and sudden self-defense situations are fought with fists, elbows and grappling techniques.

So does this mean that unless you are a taekwondo competitor, you should slack off on training your kicks? Of course not. But it does mean that if your fighting style emphasizes kicks or you just enjoy the heck out of kicking all the time, you need to spend more time working on your hand techniques. If this is hard to do in class—tuh duh!—work them when you train by yourself.

Let's begin by examining your basic hand techniques to see how you can make them better, stronger and faster. These are the bread-and-butter techniques, the ones most fighters fall back on under stress. Even if you are predominately a hand technician, it does not hurt to revisit your basics from time to time.

PUNCH

Probably every punch/kick art uses the reverse punch, though some may call it by a different name. I'm referring to that straight-line punch that is launched with your right arm when you are standing in a left-leg-forward fighting stance. This can be a powerful punch when you take advantage of your forward momentum, hip rotation, opposing action of your opposite arm and rotation of your punching fist.

Most styles execute the reverse punch similarly, with minor differences in the placement of the opposite hand, position of the rear foot and the angle of the body. Variations usually exist because in the formation of the style—whether a traditional one or a new offshoot—the founders felt the nuances added something positive to the punch. This is fine as long as everything is physiologically sound. However, variations that are a result of errors, neglect or carelessness are obviously not good. When the all-important foundation of the reverse punch becomes unsound, the punch cannot live up to it's full potential.

Instructor Rick Kirkham has spent many years analyzing the mechanics of the reverse punch. He has discovered several common errors made by fighters that dramatically reduce the effectiveness of their punches. Check the following bullets to see if any, or (heaven forbid) all, of the errors apply to your reverse punch.

- *Error:* You rotate your body and lunge forward before moving your hand, which telegraphs your attack.
- *Correction:* Your punch should lead your body lunge.

- *Error:* Flipping your elbow out to the side prevents your upper gross muscle involvement.
- *Correction:* You want to involve as many muscle groups in the strike as possible, including the muscles of your upper body. Thrust your arm out in a straight line, maintaining the point of your elbow under your arm.

- *Error:* Allowing the elbow to point upward by over rotating the fist prevents upper gross muscle involvement.
- *Correction:* To feel the difference in your strength, have your partner push against your hands when your elbow is facing upward and then again when your elbow is facing downward where it should be.

- *Error:* Locking your front knee and holding your leg straight inhibits hip motion.
- *Correction:* Bend the front knee for greater range of motion.

- *Error:* Holding your rear foot flat on the floor hinders full rotational movement of the hips.
- *Correction:* Push off with the ball of the rear foot and allow your lead foot to rotate outward slightly. Rotate your hips as far as they can go for optimum punch penetration.

- *Error:* Allowing the arm to swing out in an arc, which telegraphs your punch and reduces its speed and power.
- *Correction:* To keep your punch straight, think of rubbing your side with your arm as it extends.

- *Error:* Having one foot in front of the other hinders your ability to fully rotate your hips. This is called railroad tracking, as if both of your feet are on the same rail.
- *Correction:* Put your left foot on the left rail and your right foot on the right one.

Use the Mirror

Important

Unless you are terribly homely (you know who you are), the mirror is your friend. Since it's common for even the best martial artists to get a little sloppy from time to time, practice your reverse punch reps in front of a mirror at least once a month to see that your form is where it should be. Always remember that your body constantly seeks the easiest way to move. The moment you stop paying attention to your punching form, your elbow flips out, your shoulder lifts and your rear foot floats off the floor. Although your body may find this more comfy, it does not make for a good punch. Fight your body's natural impulse to get lazy by spending time in front of the mirror at least once a month – once a week is better – to ensure that your form is right on the money.

3 sets, 15 reps – both arms

PALM-HEEL STRIKES

I'm including the palm-heel strike as a bread-and-butter technique because more and more martial arts writers advocate using it, especially when hitting the hard and uneven surface of the head. This is a good trend because the reality of punching an attacker in the head is not the same as you see in the movies. You never see Chuck Norris's character punch a bad guy in the chops and then see Chuck jump up and down and curse as he clutches his broken hand to his chest. That has happened to me and I have seen it happen to others, too. Small hand bones versus the big head bone is a sure way to the hospital's cast room.

Look at one of your palms. Notice that it's thickly padded and the striking area is supported by your wrist and forearm. Hey, life doesn't get much better than that. It's almost as if nature wants you to hit people with it. Instructor Jerry VanCook, a strong advocate of the palm-heel strike, says that you can replace your basic hand strikes—jab, reverse, hook and uppercut—with the palm-heel strike, although you have to modify your hand position for each.

To configure your hand for the palm heel, thrust your heel forward and bend your hand back toward the top of your forearm. Squeeze your fingers together and bend them, to what extent depends on the length of your fingers. Some fighters do it just a little, while others bend them until the tips touch their palms. Bend your thumb and press it against the side of your hand. Jerry VanCook says that the most common errors a fighter makes are not bending his wrist back far enough and not tightening it just before impact. He says, "Keep your hand, wrist and arm loose as you execute your strike and then tighten it just prior to hitting the target."

Important

Although I have delivered knockout punches with my fist, I have never tried with a palm-heel strike (I did, however, knock a guy over a 50-foot embankment with a palm heel. I relate that somewhat sexually provocative story in my book *Far Beyond Defensive Tactics*). I asked VanCook about his experiences using the palm heel as a knock out strike.

"Sure, you can knock someone out with it," he says. "The striking point is a little more cushioned than bare knuckles (this varies from person to person, of course), and therefore has a little more give to it. But I think the extra power that can be generated more than makes up for this. By leaving the hand open, your body's natural instinct to tighten your biceps is avoided. This means the biceps are not working against the triceps, which are used to extend your striking arm."

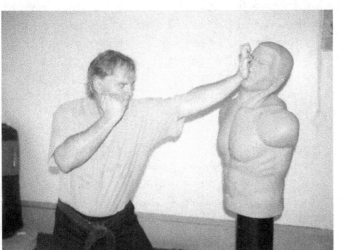

To jab with the palm-heel strike, thrust your hand straight to the target, striking with the heel of the hand.

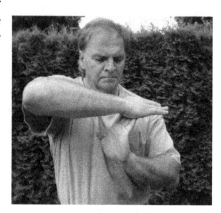

Use the palm of one hand to stretch the fingers of your other. Hold for 30 seconds.

A good way to warm up your wrists and increase their flexibility for the palm-heel strike is to stretch your fingers and hand back and hold for 30 seconds at a time. Stretch each hand a half dozen times. Begin practicing your strikes in the air.

Reverse punch palm-heel strike   Stand before your mirror, lunge forward and execute a reverse punch, substituting the palm-heel strike for the punch. Check your image to ensure that you are thrusting with your heel and pulling your fingers back enough. *2 sets, 10 reps — both sides*

Upper cut palm-heel strike   Thrust your arm upward, leading with your palm, your fingers toward the target, as if you were holding a food tray. Actually, since you need to tilt your palm in the direction of your fingers, the tray would slide forward and off your hand. This upper cut palm-heel works well against a guy bent forward, his face looking downward, say, as a result of your front kick to his groin. You step in and drive your palm up and into his nose. *2 sets, 10 reps — both sides*

Roundhouse palm-heel strike   The roundhouse palm-heel strike is delivered in a circular fashion close to your body. Keep in mind that the more you reach out with it, the greater the risk to your wrist. When hitting the head, lead with the heel of your palm and point your fingers upward. When hitting the side of the body, hold your hand so that your fingers are pointing outward instead of upward. Since the body is softer than the head, it's easy for your hand to sink in (especially when hitting a fat guy) and sprain your fingers.

2 sets, 10 reps — both hands

Now that you have a feel for the technique, move to the heavy bag and do the three basic palm-heel strikes against it. If you have not practiced these on a bag before, don't start out whacking it as hard as you can. You will have to lift your coffee cup with your elbows for a week while your wrists heal. Get the feel of each technique as to how to hit correctly, and then progressively hit the bag harder and harder.

2 sets, 10 reps — each technique, each side

Caution

BACKFIST

The backfist is a bread-and-butter technique on the tournament circuit, though it's mildly controversial among martial artists who train strictly for the street. I'm not talking about some of those bunny-pat backfist strikes that are good only for earning a point in competition, but rather a blow that can splatter a guy's face all over the clothing of onlookers. I'm not going to take up space debating its value because I think it's a great technique as long as you have the speed, power and savvy to deliver it. Here are some ways to develop those attributes.

Change Point of Origin

The point of origin is that place from where your backfist is launched, most often from an on-guard position, hands held high by the head or lower around your chest. This is fine, but it's not the only place. What if you were flipping a hair out of your eye when an opening appeared, or maybe you were bent for whatever reason with your hand near your knee. These may not be the best points of origin, but if that is the only opportunity you have—and windows of opportunity are usually short lived—take it. If the guy is nice enough to give you an opening, you need to move, and move NOW. But if you have never practiced your backfist from these odd angles, it may not be effective. It may not even occur to you to use it.

You must practice your launch from these out-of-the-norm places to ingrain the idea in your mind so you can hit with authority and confidence. Once you get proficient, you might want to deliberately put your hand in these places as a ruse to fool your opponent into thinking you are unprepared to attack. For example, after an exchange with your opponent, bend over and rest your hands on your knees as if you are winded or hurt. He moves in for the kill, and you explode up into him with your killer blow.

Backfist begins above your forehead: 3 sets, 10 reps — each hand
Backfist begins around your knee: 3 sets, 10 reps — each hand

Practice throwing your backfist from a place other than your on-guard position. For example, pretend you are rubbing your head, and then snap your backfist into the target.

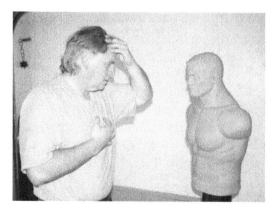

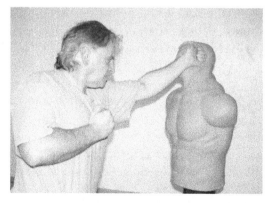

Whipping Backfist

Here is a variation of the backfist that is fast and especially powerful. Its motion is similar to a backhand slap, but in this case you strike with your big knuckles rather than the fine bones on the back of your hand (slapping with the back of the hand is not recommended and is discussed in greater detail in the section, "Slapping" page 124).

Unlike the regular backfist that shoots out in a slight arc, makes contact and then returns on the same path, the whipping backfist passes through the target and continues to complete the arc. There is no interruption in the motion with the whipping backfist. Although, I have never compared it against a regular backfist on a device that gauges impact poundage, you can clearly hear the difference on the bag, and partners holding the hand-held pads can feel the difference. I'm guessing there is greater trauma to the recipient's neck since the whip causes his head to turn with great force. I'm guessing because I have never been able to get anyone to act as a test dummy for me.

Stand before a bag in your on-guard stance, left side forward. If you have tender hands, you should wear gloves since the whip-through on the bag is a tad rough on the knuckles. Face the bag, relax your muscles and execute your backfist as you normally do. But instead of penetrating the bag with your power and then snapping your hand back, slice through it, letting your fist continue in an arc out to your side and then back to your on-guard position. If you are too far away, you will only nick the bag with your knuckles. If you are too close, your fist will land too deeply into the bag, which slows the slice. When you find that just-right-distance, your backfist will cut through the bag with a loud slapping sound. I have students who can make it sound like a rifle shot.

The whipping backfist is safest to use when you have a clear opening with little or no chance of being countered. Think of it as a coup-de-grace after you have weakened your attacker with other blows. As he staggers in place, not sure if he wants to fall, make up his mind for him with a powerful whipping backfist.

Heavy bag: 2 sets, 10 reps — both sides

To execute a whipping backfist, begin in your on-guard position. Snap out your backfist as you normally do, but instead of stopping on the target, let your fist pass through and continue out to the side.

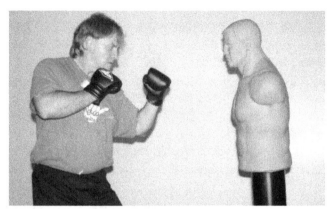

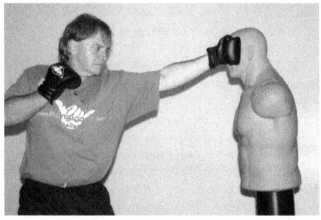

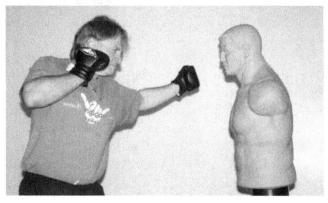

Uppercut

Although most fighting systems consider it the uppercut to be a basic hand technique, I have never been a strong advocate of it, especially the classic method of executing it. I think it's too easy to injure your hand, especially when smacking it into an assailant's jaw (I discuss the danger if striking the jaw when we talk about the palm-heel strike), or thrusting it into his abdomen. When hitting an assailant who is standing upright with an uppercut to the abdomen, your fist will simply skim up the surface without making any appreciable impact. To hurt him, the assailant's upper body must be angled just right, about 45 degrees toward you. If he is angled forward too far, however, there is risk that you will sprain your wrist.

Hitting the jaw bone or the oddly-angled upper body is not a problem if you are a boxer with taped wrists and hands while wearing heavily padded gloves. But out in the cruel street, hitting the wrong target may injure you and greatly interfere with your ability to defend yourself.

Caution

Here are two ways to use the uppercut that are relatively safe on your hands. One method concerns the angle of travel and the other way concerns the target.

Slightly Angled Uppercut

This method has been popular in tournaments since the late 1960's. It was criticized when it first appeared on the tournament scene, but when competitors began suffering broken ribs from it, it was accepted as a viable technique. It's an uppercut, though delivered with only a slight upward angle. The punching hand is thrown palm-side up and the line of trajectory is slightly upward. These two elements allow you to punch under an opponent's lead guard and blast him in the ribs, an angle that is impossible to do with a regular straight-line punch.

It's the slight, upward angle of travel that makes it hard for you to practice it alone on a bag. When you are with a workout partner, he can pull the bottom of the hanging bag back a little so that your fist hits flat and doesn't risk tweaking your wrist. But if you don't have a method of tying the bottom of the bag back when training alone, you just have to be content with practicing in the air.

Air: 3 sets, 15 reps – both sides
Bag: 3 sets, 15 reps – both sides

Hitting the Throat

The couple of times I have been struck in the throat have been unpleasant multiplied by 10. One especially bad moment was when I caught a spinning back kick to the throat, and for a few minutes I thought I was on my way to the golden dojo in the sky. I used it once as a police officer when two guys ganged up on me outside of a grocery store. When I thrust a medium-powered uppercut to the Adam's apple of the one closest to me, he crumpled to my feet as if his legs no longer existed.

Getting struck in the throat is a horrible sensation, one that is debilitating and could even be fatal. Therefore, as I've mentioned when discussing other dangerous techniques, be justified when using such serious force.

Caution

Close range technique   The uppercut is a good close-range technique, such as when you are in a clinch. When you get one hand free, pop one into your assailant's throat.

To practice this alone, move around as if you are in a clinch with someone. As you move about, repetitiously, drive uppercuts straight up in front of your face. Sometimes drop your fist about as high as your belt and thrust it upward, and other times begin with your fist in front of your chest and then thrust upward. Twist your upper body sharply with the blow and come up off your rear heel.

3 sets, 15 reps –both sides

ROUNDHOUSE PUNCH

Probably the first roundhouse punch I saw as a kid was those great big ones John Wayne launched to send his adversary head over heels through a pair of swinging saloon doors and into the dirt. I thought that was pretty cool, but the first time I tried it in a school yard fight I had to wear a heavy bandage around my sprained wrist for a couple of weeks. Today, I still have a tendency to tweak my wrists when throwing roundhouse punches at a bag.

I asked Instructor Frank Garza, who relies heavily on his roundhouse punch in full-contact matches, how he throws his. He offered two ways to punch that reduces the potential for injury. He says to deliver it close to your body, so your arm is in a stronger position and your fist is less likely to wobble. Secondly, punch with your palm side toward you so that your wrist and forearm bones are "lined up" in a stronger position than when your palm is facing downward. He says, "One other advantage of throwing hooks [roundhouse punches] this way is that when you throw them at an opponent's body, you can vary the angle slightly and cause maximum damage to the ribs. In kenpo we always try to match a vertical with a horizontal. In this case, you throw a hook punch with your palm facing you (vertical), at your opponent's ribs, which are spread horizontally to protect the lungs.

Important

"I throw several kinds of hook punches, at two different ranges, trapping and punching," Garza says. "When I throw a long-range hook, I'm really using it to get my opponent to move in the direction of my other hand so I can blast him with a cross, or perhaps even an uppercut. I don't put a lot of power in my long-range hooks because if I connect, my hand/wrist/elbow are not in a braced position. Consequently, I could hurt those joints, including my knuckles. When I throw a hook closer to my body, I'm looking to hurt the ribs or the kidney, depending on the position of my opponent."

Here is Garza's method for delivering a powerful roundhouse punch. "Take your on-guard position, left foot forward, your hands up near your chin. Then simply drop your right hand about half way down your chest and pivot your body to the left (you can dramatically increase your power if you take a slight step to the left with your left foot). Any subtle change in your body won't usually be noticed because you are throwing the punch when the opponent is close to you."

When throwing a roundhouse punch with your lead fist, turn your lead foot and your waist 90 degrees in the same direction as the punch.

If you normally do a roundhouse punch with your palm facing downward, and you have experienced pain or injury to your wrist, try punching with your palm facing you, your fist 6 to 12 inches from your body.

Start out slowly on the heavy bag until you get the feel. Once you think you are hitting correctly, progress slowly to hitting harder and harder.

Rear hand: 2 sets, 15 reps — both sides
Lead hand: 2 sets, 15 reps — both sides

Here are a couple of combinations Garza likes:

Combo 1: Throw a long-range lead hook, not with the intent to hit but rather to force your opponent to your right, where you hit him with a solid reverse punch.

Combo 2: Imagine you are in close with your opponent. Drop your right fist half way down your chest, step to the left and round-house punch his ribs.

2 sets, 15 reps – both sides

ELBOWS

When I teach arnis to new students, a typical question I get is "Can I hit him there? Will it hurt him?"The answer is yes, regardless of what target they are asking about. After all, it's soft flesh, nerves and bones being struck with a hard stick. Of course it hurts. This same truth exists with the elbow. Does it hurt to hit him there with the elbow? Yes, wherever you hit him - head, body, arms, hands, legs – it's going to hurt because the elbow is a hard bone.

Various fighting arts take different approaches to using the elbow. Instructor Frank Garza has trained in a variety of styles and explained some of the differences he has found.

"I am very fortunate to have learned so much about throwing elbows from kenpo, kali, and Muay Thai," Garza says. "I think what really differentiates the use of elbows in these three systems is the intended target. In kenpo, we throw elbows to the head or the body at different angles. In kali the elbows are used mostly to destroy limbs, biceps, triceps, and shins. In Muay Thai, I have rarely seen an elbow thrown anywhere but the face, and it's thrown in combinations like a boxer would throw a jab and cross.

"The kenpo system I learned defines the elbow strike by the particular side you have forward: right elbow or left elbow; by its method of execution: snapping elbow, thrusting elbow and whipping elbow; and by its direction of travel: upward, downward, inward, horizontal, diagonal, downward diagonal and upward diagonal. In kali, I throw elbows upward, downward, and horizontal. The Muay Thai I've studied, uses inward and spinning elbows.

"I believe if you destroy the limbs using elbow techniques from kali you won't have to worry about throwing an elbow to the face from either kenpo or Muay Thai. But then again, if you're in a bar and face to face with a guy who starts throwing a punch, hit him with two or more Muay Thai inward elbows to the face while he is cocking his hand back. That pretty much ends it.

"In Muay Thai, any time an elbow is thrown, the other hand is kept against the middle of the forehead with the thumb close to the forehead, fingers straight and pointed upward. This is done to protect the head from a counter elbow and allow the person

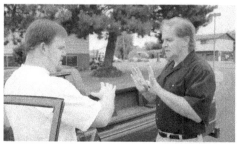

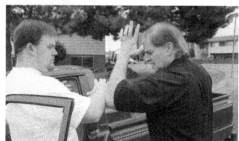

You try to calm an angry motorist but he reaches toward you. To distract him as you move in, you snap your lead elbow into the tender muscles of his upper forearm followed by a roundhouse elbow into the side of his head, Your elbow moves past his head and then snaps back into the other side of his face.

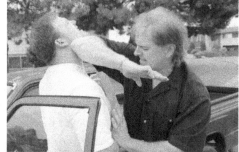

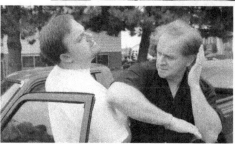

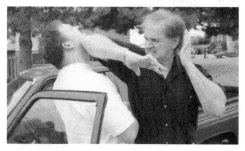

executing the technique to immediately throw another elbow from the opposite side.

"It's been my experience that it's very important to develop a flow so that if one elbow doesn't connect, the other elbow will. When you're in elbow range, throw them until you or the opponent moves to another range, be it trapping or grappling or further out in punching and kicking range; I strongly believe in flow. Muay Thai elbows flow like the limb destructions in kali."

Important

Air reps: Do reps of all the elbow strikes you know. Do one elbow strike per rep
   2 sets, 15 reps of each striking method – both sides

Bag reps: Do reps of all the elbow strikes you know. Do one elbow strike per rep
   2 sets, 15 reps of each striking method – both sides

Elbows Only Shadow Sparring

Move around as if sparring, but strike only with elbows — upward, horizontal, downward and roundhouse types. Once you are loose and flowing easily, lead off with a left jab and follow with a right elbow. Or move in with right and left elbow strikes and then punch your way out as you back off. Create combinations that work well for you and that flow smoothly in and out of range.
   3, 3-minute rounds, 1 minute rest between each round

Elbow Bag Work

Unlike the above "Bag reps" for elbows where you step in and strike and then move back, this time you move all around the bag hitting with whatever comes to mind. One way is to start in close and do combinations using only elbow strikes. You can also work from your kicking range in: kick, punch and elbow; or you can work your way out: elbow, punch and kick.
   3, 3-minute rounds, 1 minute rest periods

U PUNCH

This is sort of an odd ball technique that I stole from an old Japanese kata. My training buddies and I used to goof around and use it occasionally when sparring just to get a laugh. After a while, however, we discovered we could get it in when there was a wide-open target. I've never used it in a real situation, but I'm convinced if the opportunity was right, it would knock an attacker into the next county. It's often called the U punch.

Stand in a fighting stance with your left leg forward. As you step forward with your lead foot into forward stance, angle your upper body slightly over your lead leg as you punch out with both fists. Your right punch is basically a reverse punch and your left is a straight punch delivered palm up. To ensure that your punches are extending evenly, turn sideways to a mirror and then punch to see if your fists are stopping on the same vertical line.

You can hit with a snap punch or you can focus your power deep into the target. When snap punching, the two blows are retracted the instant they make impact, so that you can follow quickly with additional blows. With the deep focus strike, sink your fists deeply into the target and tense your chest muscles along with your arms, shoulders and abdomen. Deep focus blows are often used as a finishing technique. In both cases, imagine striking at the attacker's throat and solar plexus or his upper chest and lower abdomen.

Air punching: 3 sets, 10 reps — both sides
Heavy bag punching: 2 sets, 10 reps — both sides

Simultaneously, thrust both of your fists into the target.

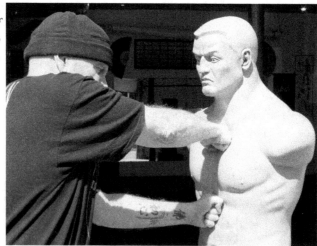

HAMMER STRIKE

The hammer strike is the Rodney Dangerfield of karate hand techniques because it gets no respect and is rarely used in sparring and drills. It should, though, because it's arguably the strongest hand technique in the fighting arts. Martial artists use it the break stones, blocks of ice and stacks of bricks.

Impact is made with the bottom of the fist, that part you pound the table with when you are angry. It's used to strike a target downward, horizontally and all angles in between. The biggest problem with the hammer is that there is nothing subtle about; an opponent can see it coming a mile away. But when you can get it in—usually as a finishing technique—its power potential can be bone crushing.

The strike's power comes from the muscles of your arms and shoulders as your fist travels on a 90- to a 180-degree arc. At first, don't deliberately try to make the blow powerful. Instead, concentrate on proper body mechanics and your speed and power will come naturally. Be cognizant of where your other arm is because the hammer fist leaves you open and vulnerable a little longer than, say, a snapping backfist. You want to retract your nonstriking fist near your head to block any surprise counters and to be in position to deliver a follow-up technique.

Training Tip

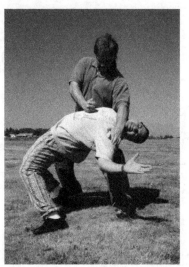

A hammer strike to the solar plexus is a great finishing blow.

Downward Strikes

Set your heavy bag on its side on a table top. It can be as high as your shoulders, as if you were striking an assailant's collar bone, or as low as your belt, as if you were striking the back of his head as he is bent over. Stand before the bag in your fighting stance, left leg forward. Cock your right fist to the side of your head and bring it down hard onto the surface of the bag. Hit with a slightly bent arm to protect your elbow from hyperextending upon impact, and be sure to retract your opposite fist. To increase your power, contract your stomach muscles and exhale sharply on impact.

3 sets, 10 reps — both sides

Backward and Upward Hammer

A less common method to hit with the hammer, but enormously effective, is to use it as a parting shot when you have been turned around and trying to break free from a clash. Say, you and your opponent exchange a flurry of punches and kicks and, in the process, you are turned sideways or your back is to him. Needless to say, this is an undesirable position for you, one you must escape from. As you do so, swing your hammer strike in an arc downward and backward, whacking your opponent in the groin. Think of it as a painful way of saying, "I'm outta here."

3 sets, 10 reps – both sides

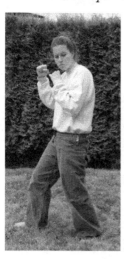

To assist in your escape when you are being held from behind, strike downward and backward into your opponent's groin.

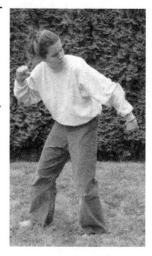

Horizontal and Diagonal Hammer Strikes

Horizontal strikes   Stand before a hanging heavy bag in your left-leg-forward fighting stance. Cock your right fist along the side of your head and bring it across your body in a horizontal fashion, striking the bag with the bottom of your fist. As before, contract your abdominal muscles and exhale on impact. Horizontal striking allows you to strike underneath your opponent's guard.

3 sets, 10 reps – both side

Diagonal strikes   To strike at an angle, position yourself before the bag, cock your fist by your head and strike downward at a 45-degree angle onto the bag. Diagonal strikes allow you to sneak in your hammer between your opponent's guard.

3 sets, 10 reps – each side

The more you train on the hammer strike, the more you find yourself using it in sparring, and the more you consider it a technique for self-defense. Use your time when training alone to perfect its delivery, and use your training time with a partner to perfect timing, distancing and various ways to get it in.

It's a powerful technique. Spend time on it.

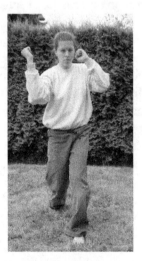

From your on-guard position, swing your hammer fist down and into your opponent's neck or ribs.

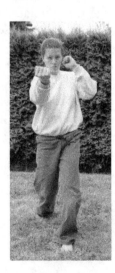

SLAPPING

I have a student who can slap the face off of a pitbull. He is so powerful that his open-hand whacks on a heavy bag can be heard a block away, and if he is slapping a hand-held bag, it's not a good time for the guy holding it. It's gruesome to imagine him slapping an assailant with it.

Slapping is a devastating hand technique that few karate fighters include in their repertoire. It's unfortunate because when executed with power, speed and proper body mechanics to the right target, it's capable of some serious hurt. It may not have the same bone-breaking and organ-damaging potential as a thrusting punch or kick, but a slap can cause acute pain, shock and unconsciousness.

As a police officer, I used it several times as a distraction device against subjects who would not release their hand from things, such as door facings, weapons or one of my prized body parts. There were also many occasions when subjects grabbed my calf or pant cuffs after I had taken them to the floor. No, they weren't admiring my attractively formed ankle, but trying to pull me down with them. Prying on their hands only tightened their grip, but a stinging slap to their ears or kidneys distracted them long enough for me to pull their hands away and slip on the silver bracelet.

While a slap is normally delivered with the palm-side of the hand, you can also strike with the back of the hand. I don't advise doing it to the face, however, because the many small and fragile bones in your hand will not stand up to the impact. Instead, turn your hand over when slapping in a backhand motion so that you make impact with your palm.

The hand configuration for slapping is quite simple. Either hold your hand flat while holding your fingers and thumb together, or cup your hand as if holding a large ball, again with your fingers and thumb pressed together. Use your cupped hand to strike an assailant's ear—which causes acute pain and possibly eardrum damage—and the flat of your hand to all other targets. Maintain a bent arm in all methods of striking so you do not hyperextend your elbow joint.

Caution
—

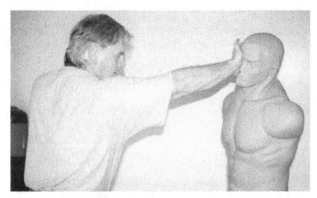

From your right-leg-forward stance, use a backhand motion to slap your right palm—moving left to right—into the side of the target, followed by a slap with your left palm.

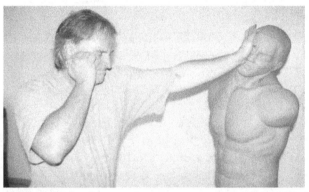

Instructor and veteran street fighter Marc MacYoung is sold on slapping in self-defense situations. He concurs that it's vital how you form your hand. "When most people talk about slaps, they think about doing them with a relaxed hand, which can pop the wrist back when impacting a face. This not only hurts you, but it wastes energy. Instead, keep your hand tight as you hit. Even if your arm is relaxed, tighten your hand (yes, this takes some muscle control, but it's worth the practice). Focus more on tightening the hand and the fingers will tend to follow. A slap done this way hits harder than most people's punches."

MacYoung likes to follow through when slapping the face as opposed to snapping his hand back. He says, "What you do with the impact is important, too. If you hit and pull back, you are not going to have nearly as much effect than if you hit and push through. If you snap your hand back, his head will bob and then snap back to reorient on you. However, when you slap and push through, you turn his head away from you."

Important

Targets for slapping:

• Face	• Stomach
• Adam's apple	• Ribs
• Side of neck	• Groin
• Upper chest	• Inner thigh

Slaps follow a circular, upward and downward direction of force. You can use your lead hand for a quick startle slap or you can use your rear one for a power slap that will make him remember the experience for a long time. Here is one way to work all the angles in one workout. Begin in your fighting stance with your left leg forward. The "left to right" and "right to left" refer to the direction your hand travels.

Lead hand
Left hand slap to ear, from left to right: 1 set, 10 reps
Left hand slap to ear, from right to left: 1 set, 10 reps
Left hand upper slap to groin: 1 set, 10 reps
Left hand downward slap to face: 1 set, 10 reps

Rear hand
Right hand slap to ear, right to left: 1 set, 10 reps
Right hand slap to ear, left to right: 1 set, 10 reps
Right hand, upper slap to groin: 1 set, 10 reps
Right hand, downward slap to face: 1 set, 10 reps

KNIFE-HAND THRUST

The knife-hand, also known as the chop, side hand and *shuto*, is typically executed in one of four ways:

1) by chambering the open hand near the ear, such as the right hand over the right ear, and then whipping it down in a circular fashion into the side of the opponent's neck,

2) by chambering the open hand over the opposite ear, say the palm of the right hand over the left ear, and whipping it in an arc to the opponent's neck,

3) by striking downward with it, such as onto an opponent's neck when he is bent over,

4) The fourth method, the knife-hand thrust is rarely used.

Let's look at how the knife-hand thrust is formed and applied against a target. Begin by assuming your fighting stance, hands up in your on-guard position, left leg forward. Thrust your right hand forward to the target, aiming with the outside edge of your open hand. Your hand and fingers must point straight upward, so that impact is made with the outside heel portion of your hand and not your fragile fingers.

Hitting the Sides of the Nose

Strike on either side of the nose on your imaginary opponent's face or the face on a manikin-type bag, or where you imagine your opponent's nose to be on a regular bag. This is a good target because the nose and the cheekbones are a somewhat softer target and less dangerous to hit than other places on the head. If you strike an assailant's mouth, for example, you can easily get cut by his teeth, which is not a good thing with all the deadly diseases going around. The forehead is a big target, but a hard one. If you don't include striking hard objects with the edge of your hand in training, it's not a good idea to start with a boney forehead.

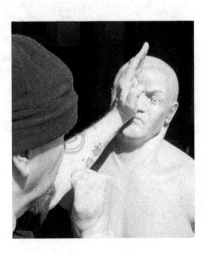

Thrust the edge of your lead hand straight into the side of your manakin's nose.

Hitting the Sides of the Neck

When thrusting into either side of the neck, you need to adjust your body a smidgen from the way you strike the side of the nose. As you launch your right hand, lean your body about 20 degrees to your right. This allows your thrust to get around his face and hit that big cord on the left side of his neck. To hit the right side, angle your body about 20 degrees to your left. A nice combination (nice to you, not to him) is to shoot your left, lead knife-hand thrust to the side of his nose, which knocks his head back, and exposes that beautiful neck of his so that you can hit it with a right knife-hand thrust.

The rear hand thrust is strongest because you incorporate your hips, waist and all the other body mechanics that blend to make your thrust powerful. Thrusting with your lead is not as strong because fewer body mechanics come into play, but it's the faster of the two.

Training Tip

Striking the air: Lead hand, 2 sets, 10 reps — both sides
Striking the air: Rear hand, 2 sets, 10 reps — both sides
Heavy bag: Lead hand, 2 sets, 10 reps — both sides
Heavy bag: Rear hand, 2 sets, 10 reps — both sides

Lean slightly to the right and thrust your knife-hand strike into the manakin's neck cord.

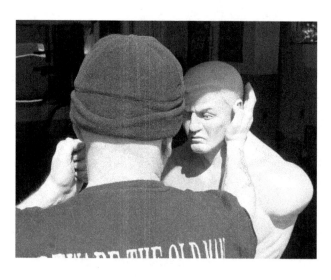

STRIKING WITH THE ARM

If you haven't used your forearm for striking, you are in for a pleasant surprise. It's easy to deliver, hard to block and causes a world of pain to the victim.

Inside and Outside Forearm Strikes

Let's call the thumb side of your forearm the "inside" and the little finger side the "outside" forearm. Both are used to deliver painful strikes to your opponent's vulnerable targets—head, neck, ribs and groin—and to less vulnerable ones like the chest, back, upper arms and thighs. While the latter targets are not as susceptible to pain and debilitation as those in the first grouping, you can still hit them to cause momentary distraction so you can get to the more vulnerable ones.

Striking with the inside of the forearm is similar to throwing a roundhouse punch and striking with the outside of the forearm is a similar motion to the backfist. When striking with either side, it's imperative that you keep your arm bent to prevent injury to your elbow joint. Here are three ways you can practice forearm strikes in the air and on a bag.

Caution

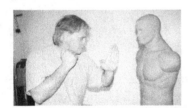

Slap aside your imaginary opponent's punch and because he is so close, counter with an outside forearm strike to his nose.

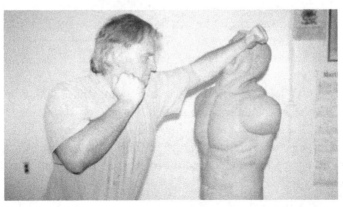

Forearm from behind   Face your imaginary opponent in your fighting stance. Step forward and drive a right reverse punch into his chest, followed by a left elbow to his ear. Whip your right arm around behind his head and snap the inside of your forearm into the back of his skull. He can't defend against the elbow because he can't see it. Work to make the combination flow smoothly.

Air: 3 sets, 10 reps – both sides
Bag: 3 sets, 10 reps – both sides

Forearm to nose   Face your imaginary opponent in your fighting stance, left leg forward. He throws a reverse punch that you slap to the right with your lead hand, but he continues to move forward, and before you can retract your blocking hand so as to backfist him, he is too close. No problem, you still have the outside of your forearm, which you ram into the point of his nose.

Air: 3 sets, 10 reps – both sides
Bag: 3 sets, 10 reps – both sides

Forearm to groin   You and your imaginary opponent are exchanging a series of blows and blocks. You lose your footing and go down on one knee in front of him. He moves in for the kill but you are too quick for him as you snap your forearm up between his legs.

Air: 3 sets, 10 reps – both sides
Bag: 3 sets, 10 reps – both sides

Hacksaw forearm   The first time I experienced this little goodie, I didn't know it had a name, but I did know that it hurt. I was training in jujitsu with Professor Tim Delgman at his San Francisco school, and he was doing a move on me in which he slid his forearm along my neck. After a half dozen reps, my baby-soft skin was bleeding from the abrasions caused by the rough sleeve of his judo gi.

When I mentioned it to him (I may have whined), he said that he was actually being kind and just barely skimming along my skin. He then did the technique the way it was supposed to be done with lots more pressure against my neck from his forearm. Not only did it hurt more, it turned me 90 degrees away from him. Since I

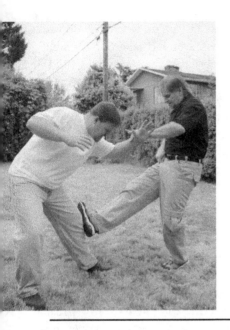

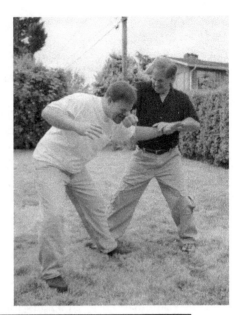

You scoop kick the assailant's closest knee, which brings his head forward. Place your right forearm against the side of his face and hacksaw your forearm forward, which twists his head hard to his right. Follow up with a claw to his face and scoop kick to his other knee.

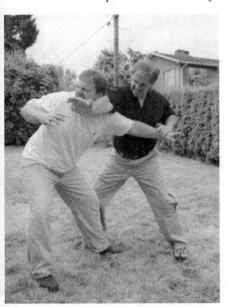

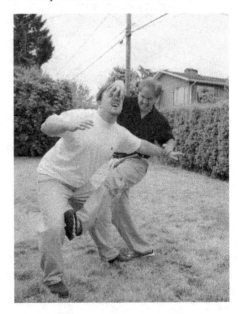

enjoyed that so much, he showed me a variation where he slid his forearm along my face. This time I spun even further around, which made it a piece of cake for him to apply a follow-up grappling hold.

The next time I saw the technique was in a book called *Indonesian Fighting Fundamentals: The Brutal Arts of the Archipelago* by Instructor Bob Orlando, who teaches an eclectic mixture of Chinese kuntao and Indonesian pentjak silat. In his system, he teaches a principle called "adhesion" where instead of knocking your opponent away from you, which gives him an opportunity to come back fighting, you remain virtually stuck to him so that you can easily finish him off with additional blows.

Important

One method of applying adhesion to an opponent is to use the forearm rub Professor Delgman used so painfully well on me. Orlando calls it "hacksaw" saying that it's characteristic of pentjak silat. In his book, he says that the hacksaw motion neither chops like an axe nor cuts like a saber. "...it saws through the target using a combination of lateral and forward motion," he writes. "[A real hacksaw] works not by simply skimming across or gliding over the object it is to cut. It presses into the object as it is pushed along."

Bob Orlando explained one method of using the hacksaw against an opponent's head. "I often use the hacksaw on my opponent's head or neck to cause his head to turn away. Rotating his head rotates his body, while a direct blow often sends him back, but with his fists and feet still trained on me. Rotating my attacker and hacking through his head, neck, or shoulders are some of the very best ways to keep him within range and under my control. I say 'my control' because he reacts pretty much the way I expect (read: dictate) him to react. By turning his ugly head, I also turn his hands and feet away from me. Moreover, I prevent him from seeing, and possibly countering what I'm going to do next. The hacksaw allows me to stick to my opponent, direct his motion, and remain in position to dissuade him from his self-destructive actions. A similar blow to the head (without the adhesion inherent in the hacksaw) may knock him down, but then I'll have to run the gauntlet of his legs to secure a similarly advantageous position."

Hacksaw is a little tricky to practice alone. You can do it on an imaginary opponent as long as you can create and maintain a clear image of his reactions to what you are doing. You can also do it on a bag to get a general feel for the sawing motion. Here is a simple combination you can practice in the air and on a bag to get you thinking of other ones.

Kick, hacksaw and knee strike the air   Face your imaginary opponent with your left leg forward. Kick his forward knee with a right scoop kick ("Scoop kick", page 54). He will react by bending slightly, or a lot, over his kicked knee, which will position his head a little closer to you. Shoot your right forearm to his face and hacksaw it along his features. The sawing motion will turn his head to his right. Cup his eyes with your right hand and thrust a left scoop kick into his other knee.
2 sets, 10 reps – both sides

Kick, hacksaw and knee strike the bag   This works best with a manikin, but you can make do with a regular hanging bag. Face the bag and kick the air as if hitting your opponent's knee. Set your foot down in front and shoot your right forearm across the face of the bag, cup it with your palm and drive a knee strike into it.
2 sets, 15 reps – both sides

LEAD HAND TECHNIQUES

Most styles deliver the uppercut, roundhouse punch, and ridgehand strike with their rear hand, meaning that when they stand with their left leg forward, they throw these techniques with their right hand. But let's say you are in a real fight or a sparring session and an opening occurs that is perfect for one of these techniques—but with your lead hand. The problem is that you never practice them with your lead, so you are either going to deliver a weak and ineffective blow, or let the opportunity pass—and a missed opportunity can be disastrous. This need not happen.

It's all about Body Mechanics

When throwing an uppercut with the rear hand, for example, twisting your waist and hips and driving off your rear foot adds power to the strike. But since these body parts are less involved when executing your lead uppercut, you must figure out how to use your body to bring as much power to the blow as you can.

Lead hand uppercut   Although there are several variations of the lead upper cut, let's discuss one that is effective in the street, one that is closer to boxing.

Begin with your left leg forward with your hands held high in an on-guard position. Since you don't have the capability to twist your hips as far as you do when using the rear arm, you have to compensate by angling your upper body. Drop your lead, left arm to the level of your belt, but keep your right arm up by the right side of your forehead guarding your face. Some pro boxers drop it even lower. In fact, Mike Tyson drops his almost to his lead knee. I don't recommend this when you first experiment with the lead uppercut because dropping it that low is one of those exceptions to the rule that works for some people—people who are experienced with the technique and who have exceptional speed.

Important

For now, drop your fist to belt level, lean your upper body slightly to the left and then fire your fist straight up. Straighten your legs slightly as you punch, so that your body lifts up a little to add momentum and body weight to the blow. A fraction of a second before impact, your upper body snaps about 45 degrees to the right. Some fighters don't turn their lead foot at all during the punch, while others rotate no more than 30 degrees to the right. Experiment to see what works best for you.

3 sets, 10 reps —each side

Lead hand roundhouse   This is a boxing technique, or rather, it used to be only a boxing technique. But now, more and more karate fighters are discovering it's power, sneakiness and versatility. It's perfect for getting around an opponent's guard. He thinks he has been clobbered from out of the blue, since the punch came from outside of his peripheral vision. Although the stronger roundhouse punch is thrown with the rear arm, the lead round can be surprisingly powerful when executed with proper body mechanics.

Assume your left-leg-forward fighting stance and think "90," which means that at the conclusion of your left, lead-arm roundhouse, your arm will be positioned at a 90 degree angle, your lead foot will be twisted 90 degrees to the right and your upper body will be twisted 90 degrees to the right. Here is how you get there:

From your on-guard position, launch your lead fist first, followed a fraction of a second later by a dynamic twist of your lead foot to the right and a snap of your hips, which twists your upper body to the right. Your right fist retracts to the side of your head. Now, check yourself out. If your arm, lead foot and hips are all 90 degrees to the right, you did it correctly.

Air punches: 3 sets, 10 reps — both arms
Bag punches: 3 sets, 10 reps — both arms

Lead ridgehand   The rear hand ridgehand (say that five times in a row real fast) strike is a popular tournament technique that is usually executed by leaping across the ring and launching it in sort of a wild, flailing motion. Although, there are few self-defense situations where you would execute it as tournament competitors do, there are other, safer ways to use the ridgehand that are devastating, especially when striking the neck. I used it once to hit a guy in the neck in a real fight and the impact caused him to do a partial cartwheel off his motorcycle. I don't know who was more surprised, him or me.

Although the rear hand ridgehand strike is the strongest and most often used, let's consider doing it with the lead hand.

The body mechanics of the lead ridgehand are similar to the way the lead roundhouse punch is thrown. For example, say the attacker is chest to chest with you in a clinch. Launch your ridgehand by whipping it in an arc behind his head and then snapping it into the back of his neck or skull. He didn't see a thing and can't begin to imagine why he is crumpling to the ground. It's more common, however, to throw it with a slightly bent arm (hitting with a straight arm can be painfully traumatic to your elbow joint). Since your arm is extended most of the way out, you can strike him from further away than with your roundhouse punch. For added power, lean a little in the direction of the strike and rotate your upper body about 30 degrees, also in the same direction.

Strike with your palm down and thumb tucked across your palm so that impact is made with the outside bone of your pointer finger. Striking with your hand flat (parallel to the floor) can be injurious to that bone, so tilt the striking part of your hand downward about 45 degrees.

Caution

Air strikes: 2 sets, 10 reps — each side
Bag strikes: 2 sets, 10 reps — each side

Here is a sneaky way to get in a ridgehand when in close. Shoot your hand past your opponent's head and then snap your ridgehand into the back of his neck.

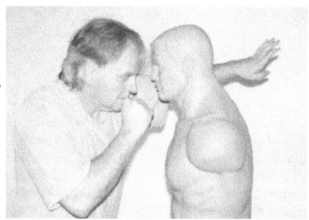

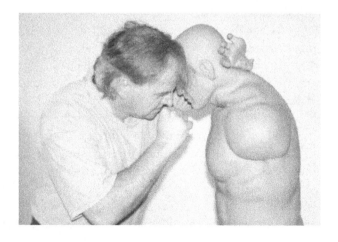

Let's take a look at a few exercises you can do when training alone that when practiced regularly, will increase the power and speed of your punches, strikes and grabs. I have included these particular exercises for two reasons: They are not the same old ones you see in every martial arts magazine and book and, most importantly, they work.

RAW LIMB PUNCHING

"Raw limb" is a term that describes techniques where only the attacking limb moves without the assistance of your body. Let's examine it as to how you throw your straight punch while standing in a natural stance. Since your body is motionless and you move only your arm, the exercise is a no brainer. You simply extend your arm and bring it back. Here is how you do it and why it's so good for you.

Stand in front of a mirror, your feet together, arms hanging down at your sides. Lift your right fist along your side, as high as your solar plexus, allowing your left arm to hang limply at your side throughout the technique. The motion is to simply extend your fist straight out, shoulder high with the usual fist rotation, and then return it to its starting position. Remember that the punch involves only your arm without even a little help from your body.

Variations

There are two variations of the raw limb punch. One is to punch out as fast as you can and snap it back as fast as you can. You didn't move your body, did you? The second variation is to punch out fast, but focus your strength for one second at full extension before you pull it back. Focus means to tense your fist, shoulders, chest and abdominal muscles. Consider the first variation a snap punch and the second one a power punch.

Raw limb punching is a great exercise to isolate the action of the punching arm. You don't have to think about stepping in, snapping your hips or retracting your other arm. You only have to extend the arm to the target. As you push to punch faster and faster, be careful not to lockout at full extension. You want to use that elbow for a few more years.

Snap back punch: 1 set, 15 reps — each side
One second focus punch: 1 set, 15 reps — each side

PUNCHING WITH MINIMUM BODY MECHANICS

Perhaps the fastest hand technique, though far from the strongest, is one that uses only minimum help from your body. The concept is similar to Raw Limb Punching except this is not an exercise but rather an actual way of delivering a technique to an opponent. It's for those times when the target presents itself and is close enough for you to hit it without taking a step. You simply lash out with your jab, backfist or reverse punch, using a minimum of movement from your shoulders and hips.

Stand before a heavy bag or a double-end bag in your neutral stance, as if you were standing in line at the movies. Stand close enough so that you don't need to step and then lash out with your technique, turning your shoulder and hips a little with the blow. Since you can't generate much power here, at least not as much as when you use all of your body mechanics, think in terms of hitting your imaginary opponent's eye, ear, nose, throat and groin, targets that don't require a lot of power to get results.

Push for speed.

On the bag: 2 sets, 10 reps, each technique – both sides

CHAIR PUNCHING

This is a fun way to do punching reps that works your legs as well as your arms. It's also practical in that you might be on a bus and have to spring off your seat and paste a guy in the chops when he refuses to turn down his boom box (I'm kidding, I'm kidding). But your ability to get out of a seat fast is important, so here is one way to do it and incorporate a punch.

Sit in your chair in a way that is normal for you, and then spring forward as fast as you can into a left-leg-forward stance and execute a right reverse punch. Recover, sit back down and do it again. Figure out what you need to do to move fast, and then push yourself to go faster and faster.

2 sets, 15 reps — each side

AIR GRABBING

This is a great series of exercises that will develop the muscles in your hands and forearms to facilitate your punching and blocking, and improve your speed and strength for grabbing. The exercises are easy to do and you will be rewarded with a great muscle pump and a burning ache in your forearms. Think of the ache as a positive indication that you are working the muscles correctly.

If you are going to do a lot of heavy bag work during your solo session, it's a good idea to do the air grabbing exercises afterwards. When you do them prior to hitting the bag, your fatigued forearms and wrists may buckle under the hard, slamming impact.

Close fist grab Extend both arms in front of you, palms out and fingers splayed. Close your fingers into a fist as quickly as you can and then open them to the fingers-splayed position.

180 reps in 30 seconds — gradually increase the reps (Some experts can do 300 reps in 30 seconds)

Caution

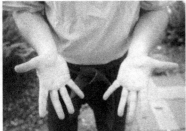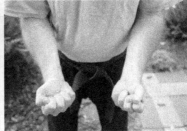

Fingers to thumb grab   Extend both arms in front of you, palms forward and fingers splayed. As quickly as you can, touch your four fingers to your thumb and then back open to the fingers-splayed position.

180 reps in 30 seconds — gradually increase the reps

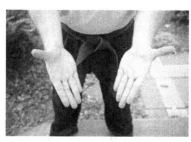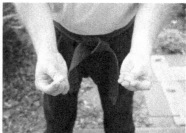

Rolling fingers grab   Extend both arms in front of you, palms forward and fingers splayed. Make a fist as in Grab 1, but begin by closing your little fingers, ring fingers, middle fingers, pointer fingers and thumbs, in that order. Return to the fingers- splayed position.

150 reps in 30 seconds – gradually increase the reps

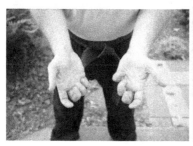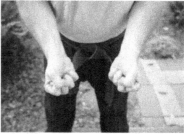

Finger slap grabs Extend both arms in front of you, palms forward and fingers splayed. Slap your fingers against the heel of your hand as your thumb remains pointing out to the side, and then open them back to the fingers splayed position. This is the easiest grab to do, so I always do it last when my hands are tired from the others.

180 reps in 30 seconds – gradually increase the reps

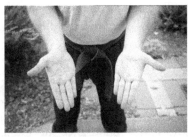 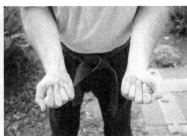

Begin by doing only one set of each grab. As you get stronger and faster, add one set to the first exercise, and then in a week or two, add another set to the second exercise, and so on. Usually, two sets each of the four grabs are plenty, especially since you are pushing for speed.

HAND TECHNIQUES WITH WEIGHTS

I'm just going to touch on the subject of using progressive resistance since I discussed it at length in my books *Power Karate: How to Develop Explosive Punches, Kicks, Blocks, and Grappling* and *Speed Training: How to Develop Your Maximum Speed for Martial Arts.*

Practicing your hand techniques while holding dumbbells gets results because you work the very muscles you want to strengthen. Although the bench press is a longtime favorite among weight lifters and is an excellent exercise for developing tremendous upper body power, it only indirectly develops punching power. Repetitiously punching with dumbbells, however, goes right to the specific muscles you want to target, including muscles involved in directions of force

Workout
Tip

other than linear, such as diagonal for the backfist, upward for the uppercut and circular for the roundhouse punch.

Although some trainers teach shadow sparring while holding weights, I don't believe this is a good way to train. If you were lifting weights for general purposes, would you do one bench press rep, three curls with just one arm, two squats, one triceps press and a couple of shoulder presses? Of course not, because it would not be productive. It's for this same reason that it's not productive to shadow spar with weights. You shuffle around and throw only one jab, and a moment later a single backfist, followed by a double punch. You continue in this erratic fashion for your entire shadow sparring session. Some techniques get more reps than others and one arm may get more reps. This is not systematic and being systematic is what encourages strength gain when doing resistance exercises. Shadow sparring is a valuable training tool for developing rhythm, fluidity of movement, balance, coordination, endurance and so on. But if you are trying to develop muscle, train systematically and skip shadow sparring with weights.

Here are some important DON'TS when lifting weights to improve your martial arts techniques.

Caution

- Don't use extremely heavy weights
- Don't punch or strike fast
- Don't snap your techniques
- Don't lock your elbow at full extension
- Don't drop the weight on your toes

Those are the don'ts. Here is a quick glance at how you should do it. Your objective here is not to be a powerlifter or a hardcore bodybuilder (you don't want to have to wear those skimpy posing trunks, do you?), but to simply add resistance to the movements to build power and increase your speed. It's a nice side benefit if you develop some visible muscle from these (wear a tank top), but your primary goal is to develop basic hand techniques that are so fast and powerful that they can knock the head off a statue.

You don't need to use tremendous weight, but a poundage that allows you to move at about 1/4 of your regular speed. As always, be careful to not forcefully lock out your elbow to full extension.

The Jab

Standing jab   Hold a dumbbell in each hand. From your fighting stance, extend your lead arm out in a jab and return it to your on-guard position. If your style jabs with the fist thumb-side up, do it that way with the dumbbell. If you normally rotate your fist, you should rotate the weight. Your other hand should retract on each rep the same way you usually do. Punch at 1/4 speed.

3 sets, 10 reps — both sides

Lying jab   Lie on your back on a bench or an exercise ball, holding a dumbbell in only your right hand. Position the dumbbell so that it's by your chin, as if you were jabbing in a standing position. Angle your body to the left and jab straight upward, being careful not to snap your elbow joint.

3 sets, 10 reps — both sides

Lie on a bench or an exercise ball and thrust a dumbbell from your chin straight up as if throwing a jab.

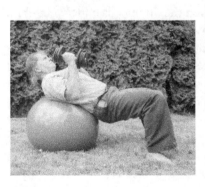
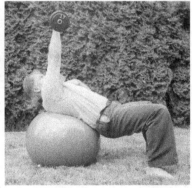

Reverse Punch

Standing reverse punch: Hold a dumbbell in each hand and from your fighting stance, lunge forward with your lead foot and execute a reverse punch. Retract your opposite hand, but be careful not to bop yourself in the head with the weight (been there, done that) then return to your on-guard position. Punch at 1/4 speed.
3 sets, 10 reps — both sides

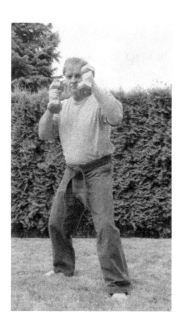 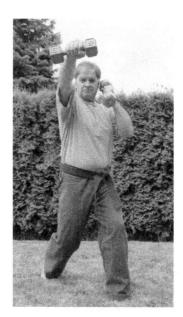

Lying reverse punch: Lie on your back on a bench, holding a dumbbell in each hand. Position the dumbbells under your chin, about 10 inches off your upper chest. The position is roughly the way you would hold your hands in your on-guard position while standing. At 1/4 speed, execute a right punch straight up as you retract your left hand slightly toward your left side and then return both hands to your starting position. Rotate your punch as you normally do.
3 sets, 10 reps — both sides

Backfist

Bungee cord   The same bungee cords you use for developing your kicks are used in this exercise. Secure an end of the cord to a post, tree or pole so that it's about as high as your shoulders. Secure the other end to your wrist or loop it around your palm, and make a fist. You may have to stand a little more sideways in your fighting stance than you normally do in order to accommodate the cord. Move back until it becomes taught and then launch your backfist at 1/4 your normal speed.

3 sets, 15 reps – both sides

The cable backfists and the dumbbell backfists listed below are also found in my book *Speed Training*. I apologize if I'm being redundant, but I've added them here because they work the exact muscles involved in the backfist and they can be added easily to your weight lifting routine as one of your exercises for your triceps.

Cable backfists   If you belong to a health club or you have cables in your home gym, include this exercise in your arm work-out. Ideally, your cable should be shoulder high, but if your system begins at floor level or a place higher than your head, you can still do the exercise. Position yourself as you did with the bungee cord and do your backfists.

3 sets, 15 reps – both sides

Dumbbell backfists   Lie on the floor on your left side and pick up a dumbbell with your right hand. Extend your left arm along the floor for balance and lean your body in that direction. Begin with the dumbbell just below your chin and extend it upward in a backfist motion. I don't think it's healthy for your elbows to lower the weight all the way back to your chin area, but if the weight is light and you have healthy joints, it's your decision to make. However, if the weight is heavy enough that you grunt, lower the weight only to a point where your forearm is horizontal with the floor. Perform your reps at about 1/4 your backfisting speed and never snap your elbow joint at the end.

3 sets, 10 reps – both sides

Roundhouse punch   Pick up a dumbbell in each hand and assume your fighting stance. Without stepping forward, throw a rear-hand roundhouse punch at a slight upward angle and be sure to retract your opposite hand. The upward angle increases the resistance against your muscles. Return your punching hand to your on-guard position and punch again. Do rear hand roundhouses and lead hand roundhouses.

Lead hand: 3 sets, 10 reps – both arms
Rear hand: 3 sets, 10 reps – both arms

Training Tip

Uppercut   Hold a dumbbell in each hand and assume your fighting stance. Drop your striking fist a little lower than you normally do so that you get a greater range of motion with the weight. Step forward and execute your uppercut punch at 1/4 your normal speed, extending it a few inches higher than you normally do. Be sure to retract your opposite hand.

3 sets, 10 reps – each hand

There are many other weight exercises you can do to improve your hand techniques, and I encourage you to seek them out. The primary requirement is that they follow the same track as the movement you want to strengthen. Always use caution as you move at about 1/4 of your normal speed and never forcefully lock out your elbow joints.

Okay, now that you have bulging muscles, let's get them moving faster than ever before with some great exercises that increase your speed.

SPEED DRILL

This is one of those drills that works so amazingly well that before doing it, you glance furtively left and right, like a young shoplifter in a store's toy section. This is because you want to keep this one to yourself, especially from any potential opponents. The beauty of this is that you can easily apply it to any punch, kick or block. For now, though, let's examine how you do it with your reverse punch. Make sure no one is watching . . . and let's begin.

First Half

Stand before a mirror and assume your fighting stance, left leg forward, fists near your chin. You are going to do a right hand reverse punch as you step forward with your lead foot, but you are going to do it in two increments. In the first half of the movement, exhale sharply as you snap your fist halfway out and retract your other hand halfway to your ear. Your right hip snaps around and your rear foot begins to come up on the ball. That is as far as you go, and then return to the beginning position. As you practice repetitiously, your objective is to push yourself to move faster and faster. This is a good one to employ the startle reflex ("Developing Explosiveness", page 158).

3 sets, 10 reps - both sides

Second Half

For the second half of the drill, begin where the first half ended. To punch fast from this point is challenging because you don't have the benefit of the momentum that normally builds from the beginning of the move. But that is why this is so good for you, because it forces you to combine your physical and mental facilities to drive yourself to move faster and faster each rep. Begin with your right fist half way out, your left fist almost to your left ear, your hips twisted almost all the way forward and your rear foot part way up. Say "Go!" in your mind and explode. As your punching fist rips forward, lunge with your left foot, snap your left fist all the way back to your ear, snap your hips the rest of the way around and drive off the ball of your rear foot. Rip! Snap! Drive! Fast!

3 sets, 10 reps - both sides

Half-rep kicking   Half reps with kicks are done the same as you did with your hand techniques.

First half: Snap your leg half way out into the kick and stop. Be sure to incorporate proper hip rotation and any movement required with your shoulders for the particular kick you are working. Push yourself for maximum speed and thrust and don't hold back.

3 sets, 10 reps for each type of kick – both sides

Second half: Beginning at the half way position, thrust or snap your kick the rest of the way out. Be sure to finish your hip rotation and any action with your shoulders. Be careful, it's easy to lock out your knees painfully when practicing second-half kicking. *3 sets, 10 reps for each type of kick – both sides*

As you prepare to launch yourself in either the first or last half of the punch or kick, maintain a physical state of relaxed readiness. It's not about moving forward quickly, but rather *exploding* forward as if startled. If it helps, be your own starter pistol and say "Bam!" each time you punch. The drill is all about speed, so don't hold back.

Partial-rep Shadow Sparring

This is a fun, result-producing speed exercise that saves your elbow and knee joints because you are not extending all the way out. Begin shadow sparring as you normally do, but extend only 6 to 10 inches with your hand techniques and 12 to 18 inches with your kicks. There is no need to extend any farther than that because you are working only the explosive first few inches of your techniques.

Here is why this works. Since you are only extending part way, your techniques are much faster than when you fully extend them. In just a few workouts, your neuromuscular system adapts to the greater speed, which then transfers to your fully-extended techniques. In other words, after doing the partial-rep sparring exercise for a while, you will throw fully extended punches at the same speed as do your partials. How cool is that?
Shadow spar, 10 minutes

Important

Overspeed Punching

I stole this idea from the excellent book *Warrior Speed* written by my friend Ted Weimann. The training concept of overspeed is to force your neuromuscular system, in this case the system of your punching arm, to move faster than it can on its own. Perhaps you have heard of track competitors who train by running sprints down hills or by being pulled by a car. The idea is to force these athletes to run just a tad faster than they can on their own (let's hope the driver is paying attention and not grooving to the sounds on the stereo).

Ted says that you can use this same concept with bungee cords to work your punches. He says to use two cords, one attached to each wrist so you can work combinations, but if you have only one cord, you can work one arm at a time. Attach one cord to your right wrist and back away from the pole, wall or whatever you have the cord secured to until you feel a slight pull on your arm. Assume your forward stance, left leg forward, and hold your arms up in your on-guard position.

Don't punch yet! First, I want to warn you to not let the cord force your arm into hyperextension. Always, and I mean always, stop your arm just short of lockout. Okay, I'm done doing my mother thing; you can punch now.

There is no need to move your feet forward since you are already in your forward stance. Punch straight out, allowing the cord to pull your arm faster than you normally punch. Be sure to retract your other hand and twist your hips into the blow. This also works well for other straight-line techniques, such as jabs and backfists, but circular ones, such as the roundhouse and ridge hand, are virtually impossible to do with the cord.

Workout
Tip

I asked Ted if he had learned any more about overspeed since he had written the book. "There is not much to add regarding overspeed training," he said. "It's been around for about 25 years but has only became popular in the early 1990's. I don't know of any scientific studies to prove it; it's only a theory."

Well, the white coats may not be making it official, but word of mouth from top athletes is that it works. Give it a try, but be careful with your elbows.

2 sets, 10 reps — both sides

5

SPARRING COMBINATIONS

Although the primary slant of all of my books is how to train to survive a street encounter, I don't want to completely ignore fighters who enjoy competition. Therefore, I have provided you with a large collection of proven combinations that are applicable for tournament sparring. Your assignment is to practice them when training alone, and push yourself to execute them faster and faster while maintaining good form and balance. When you feel comfortable with them, use a live partner to figure out how to get your well-honed techniques into a moving target(s).

There are lots of combinations here that you will like and no doubt lots that you will not. You cannot always determine which is which by just looking at the list, so I encourage you to give each an honest try. Think of your repetition practice as similar to rubbing sandpaper on a rough piece of wood. The more you rub, the smoother the wood gets. Likewise, the more you practice reps, the smoother your movements become.

Consider ways to make tournament techniques street applicable.

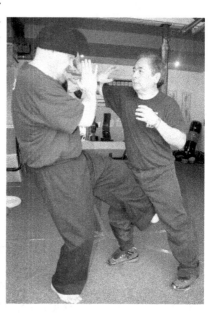

If you are not interested in tournament competition, you can use these combinations as a starting point for creating realistic, offensive attacks. You can cut and paste, combining part of one combination with another, or you can keep those combinations you feel are street realistic and eliminate those you deem too fancy or too complicated. Once you get the combination the way you want it, or find some that you like, practice them repetitively.

Remember. Repetition is your friend.

Workout Tip

It's a good idea to practice the combination from both sides: left-leg-forward fighting stance and then right-leg-forward fighting stance. Not only does this lead to balanced development, but you also learn which is best for a particular combination. Often, what you think is going to be your favorite side turns out not to be, and vice versa. You won't know, though, unless you practice on both sides many, many times.

Begin all of these with your left leg forward. Do 2 sets of 10 reps on both sides, but don't do all of the combinations listed here in one workout because you will die. Pick only two or three for each session and through trial, error and elimination, you will have a repertoire of 5-10 combinations that are yours.

- Backfist, reverse punch, roundhouse with front leg, reverse punch
- Jab, reverse punch, rear leg front kick
- Jab, reverse punch, outside crescent with lead leg
- Roundhouse kick with lead leg, reverse punch, front kick with rear leg
- Front kick with lead leg to groin, spin back kick, backfist, reverse punch
- Roundhouse with lead leg to deliberately miss, spinning rear leg hook kick, reverse punch
- Front kick with lead leg, spinning back kick, reverse punch
- Slap kick with front leg to groin, front kick with rear leg, reverse punch
- Roundhouse with front leg to groin, jab, reverse punch
- Roundhouse with front leg to face, backfist, upper cut
- Side kick, backfist, reverse punch
- Backfist, side kick with lead leg, backfist, reverse punch
- Double reverse punch, lead ridge hand
- Jab, backfist with same hand, reverse punch
- Front kick with lead leg, front kick with rear leg, set down in front and roundhouse kick with same leg
- Backfist, turning back kick, backfist, reverse punch
- Jump front kick with lead leg, backfist, reverse punch, lead ridge hand
- Jab, sweep with lead leg, reverse punch
- Side kick with lead leg, turning back kick, reverse punch
- Right punch, left punch, slap kick groin with lead leg, turning hook kick
- Jab, sweep with lead leg, turning hook kick
- Palm fake to face, leg sweep, turning back kick
- Driving reverse punch, pursue with a leadleg front kick, front kick with rear leg, reverse punch
- Jump in back fist, spinning hook kick
- Turning back kick, roundhouse kick with either leg
- Lead side kick, lead hook kick, back fist, reverse punch

- Jab, jab, roundhouse to groin with lead leg, roundhouse to head with lead leg
- Lead hook punch, rear hand upper cut to middle, turning hook kick
- Jumping lead leg roundhouse kick, front kick with real leg
- Lead leg sweep fake, spinning hook kick with rear leg
- Reverse punch to groin, lead ridgehand to neck
- Outside crescent with lead leg, rear leg inside crescent
- Backfist, rear ridgehand
- Roundhouse with rear leg and set down in front, rear leg sweep, backfist
- Sweep with rear leg set in front, outside crescent with same leg, rear roundhouse kick, reverse punch
- Lead jab, lead jab, rear hook punch, lead jab
- Side kick with rear leg, turning back kick, back fist, reverse punch
- Axe kick with either leg and set down in front, reverse punch
- Spinning hook kick with rear leg and set down in front, side kick with same leg, straight back kick with same leg
- Arm grab with lead arm and jerk, reverse punch
- Jumping back fist, backfist again upon landing
- Fake reverse punch, fake reverse punch, fake reverse punch followed immediately with a lead roundhouse kick (broken rhythm)
- Fake front hip motion as if throwing a roundhouse kick, repeat, repeat and immediately backfist (broken rhythm)
- Sweep with lead heel, backfist
- Hook kick with lead leg to miss, roundhouse with same leg, reverse punch
- Spinning hook with rear leg to sweep, roundhouse kick with rear leg
- Fake sweep with lead heel, roundhouse kick with same leg
- Fake reverse punch, backfist with same hand

- Backfist, spinning crescent with rear leg
- Jumping reverse punch, reverse punch again as you land
- Roundhouse to face with lead leg, roundhouse to abdomen with same leg, roundhouse to groin with same leg

You can add to or subtract from these as you see fit. Insert your favorite techniques into whatever combination you want or put in ones that you want to improve. There are no blocks in this list because the techniques are strictly offense. Feel free, though, to insert them wherever you see fit.

6

ODDS & ENDS WORKOUT

I call this chapter "Odds and Ends" for two reasons: One, I couldn't think of a better title. Two, the exercises and techniques presented here don't fit easily into the other chapters. That doesn't mean they are not beneficial. Nothing could be further from the truth. They are, however, a little off beat, and as such, they may not get as much training time in class as the more standard exercises and techniques. In fact, in some schools they don't get any exposure. Nonetheless, they are valuable, and I encourage you to examine them when training alone.

DIRTY SOCK DRILL

This reminds me of some of those training scenes in those horribly dubbed old Hong Kong movies from back in the 1970s and 1980s. The hero, training to avenge some wrong to his family, his school or his master, hangs bags of rice or overripe melons from a beam. He then moves about the swinging objects, punching, kicking and getting bopped in the head with them. As time passes, he is able to hit each one perfectly, exploding them in a shower of rice and melon guts. Well, these are modern times now. Today you hang old, smelly socks from the ceiling.

This drill was suggested by Instructor Daniel Alix who says it's a great way to train your reflexes, punches, strikes, body evasion and footwork. Here is how Alix describes the set up and the drill: "Fill a bunch of socks with dried beans (or rocks if you're hard-core), and tie them to the ends of a light rope. You need a room with a drop-ceiling or beams, so you can hang the socks from them. You should be surrounded by three to five menacing socks, some hanging face high and others chest high. The farther apart they are, the easier the exercise; the closer they are, the harder.

"Punch one and get out of its way before it swings back. As you move away, punch or kick another one. Get out of it's way and punch or kick another. To avoid getting hit by the swinging socks, you can work on ducking, sidestepping as you hit them, and leaning away as you hit them again. If one of them hits you, consider that you have been tagged by your opponent, in this case, a dirty sock. It's a great exercise for your footwork and it's great for your hands and feet, too, especially if you use a big variety of blows. Some fighters use many targets, but I think it turns into a game of tag if there's more than five."

Use your imagination with this drill and develop a variety of exercises with it. Use especially smelly socks as an incentive for you to move your head fast.

DEVELOPING EXPLOSIVENESS

It's 2:00 a.m. and a noise awakens you. Was it a dream or .. . There it is again. A thump. It's coming from the hall that leads from your bedroom to the living room. You slip out of bed, feeling vulnerable in your Mickey Mouse boxer shorts. Deciding that darkness is your friend, you do not turn on your night stand light. You peer out the door into the dark hallway. It's empty.

You creep along the wall, past the pictures of the family and that big picture of you and that shiny tournament trophy. Just as you approach the bathroom—that black, gaping doorway to your right—a giant figure, dressed like Hooded Death, steps out from the room and into your path.

In a thundering heartbeat, every muscle in your body jerks rigid and your stomach slams into your throat so hard you manage only a breathy, "Agh!"

You just experienced a startle reflex. Sometimes it paralyzes you, sometimes it makes you jump a foot in the air and other times it causes you to reflexively snap out your arm.

Case in point: While in the army, I was stationed for a year in the Florida Everglades, a place that can only be described as creepy, with its bugs, snakes, alligators and UFO's (yes, UFOs. But that story is for another book). One night I was walking through the dark when a buddy, a good-looking guy who had made a hit, rock and roll record before Uncle Sam got him, sprung from the shadows for no other reason than to scare the doggy doo out of me. Well, it did do that, so much so that I yelped and reflexively whipped a roundhouse kick right into his pretty face.

His movie star looks and my hard-tipped combat boot were not a good mix. The welt, scab and swelling eventually faded, but for a while there he thought his singing career was over. I don't know if he made any other records, but I do know that while we served our country in the Everglades, he never again jumped out of the creepy darkness at me.

I didn't kick him on purpose. It was a startle reflex that exploded before I knew it. Actually, kicking when startled is unusual; people usually react with their hands in some way. They reach out to grab, hit, slap or they just cover their face. Apparently, I reacted with a kick because I had been training in karate so much (there is nothing else to do in the Everglades except be on guard for every creepy, crawly critter in existence).

Approximating the Startle Reflex

What really amazed me about this incident, besides what a big baby the guy was about getting his face kicked in, was how my foot just exploded up and into his mug. It was fast, at least fast for me, powerful and explosive. I had always worked on speed and power just as all martial artists do, but the explosiveness was something I hadn't trained for. But explode it did. I concluded that the elements of speed, power, timing, distancing and reflex all coming together at one moment was the result of my startle reflex.

Bruce Lee's extraordinary backfist is probably the best example of explosiveness that most of us have seen. Remember that famous scene in *Enter the Dragon* when Lee faces off with Bob Wall, the character with the face scar? They squared off with their lead forearms touching (not recommended in real life), and then there was a moment of silent pause. Then—Whack! Bruce Lee's backfist exploded into Wall's face so fast that it was nearly imperceptible. Everything came together in that move—speed, power, distancing and timing—like a stick of dynamite.

You can do this, too, but you need to have all of the following qualities in place. You won't develop all this by next Thursday, but with effort you will, in time, reach your potential.

- You need to have exceptional speed of movement and speed of perception.
- You need to have power that is developed from performing thousands of repetitions.
- You need to possess an understanding of timing, that is, you need to know exactly when to hit an opening and do so without thought – to do it with total reflex.
- You need to be at the right distance from the target. The closer the better, though I know some fighters who can explode across five feet of space. If you are not one of these rare fighters, then start within hitting range.

To activate your startle reflex by yourself, you need to bring out an internal quality that is a little hard to put into words. For lack of a better term, let's call it "psyche," a mental state you go into briefly to bring on that same, gut tensing sensation that erupted in your body when Mr. Hooded Death stepped out of your bathroom. When you are able to do this, and it only lasts a second, your technique will explode.

Bringing on the psyche   Stand before a mirror and assume your fighting stance. You need to be relaxed with just a bit of tension, sort of like a partially coiled spring. Burn your eyes into your reflection's forehead and deliberately increase the speed of your breathing as if you were anxiously poised on the starting blocks awaiting the bang of the starter pistol.

Bam! Explode forward with your backfist, without thought. Don't go, "1, 2, 3," or say something like, "Get ready, set ... go." Instead, catch yourself by surprise. You are waiting ...Waiting .. . *Boom!*

While you may have developed good speed and power during your training career, your ability to explode will increase these qualities twofold. It's easier to develop explosiveness with a live training partner, but when training alone, you need to develop the correct psyche.

3 sets, 10 reps – both sides

YOUR INITIAL TAKEOFF

Imagine a truck parked at the curb with its motor idling. A moment later, it accelerates away into traffic, reaching a speed of 25 mph. Now, picture that same truck, but this time, see it as it approaches you at 20 mph, and then accelerates to 25 mph as it gets even with you. Which scenario would it be easier for you to see the truck's acceleration? Clearly the first one. This is because it's far easier to see motion that comes from a static place than it is to see motion that comes from motion. The same is true when you attack.

Important

Camouflage Movement within Movement

Assume your fighting stance and, remembering the truck scenario, begin moving about. If you favor deep, kata-like stances, you may have trouble moving and will tire quickly. To move with fluidity, deceptiveness and speed, you have to stand higher (similar to a boxer's stance) with your feet closer together, roughly 12-18 inches depending on your height. Keep them moving: Sometimes bounce on the balls of your feet, other times stay flatfooted and quickly switch from left foot forward to right foot forward and back.

Sometimes bring your feet together for a fraction of a second and then move them away from each other. There is no fixed pattern: just stay in motion.

1 set, 5 minutes

Condition your Opponent

Keep your guard up; you can't fake with your arms hanging limply along your sides, nor can you attack from there without telegraphing. Move your arms around, throw short fakes with your fists, jerk your shoulders forward and snap your hips as if you are going to kick. Your purpose is to evaluate your opponent's response to you as you camouflage your real attack within your movement.

If you are going to attack with a backfist, one way to set it up is to include a couple of fake ones to "condition" your opponent to what your attack looks like in its beginning stage. If you only throw out a few fake reverse punches and then suddenly attack with a backfist, your opponent would easily decipher the difference. To condition your opponent, use a pattern such as this: reverse punch fake, reverse punch fake, fake backfist, fake backfist, reverse punch fake and then a real backfist as the fake reverse punch retracts.

Partners

2 sets, 10 reps of each camouflaged technique – both sides

Move your Attack First

Begin your hand attack by moving your hand first. If you move your body first, your opponent may not know which attack you are going to do, but he knows for sure that you are coming. Move the smaller and faster body part first, followed by the rest of your body. Try it with the backfist.

3 sets, 10 reps - both sides

Mirror Time

Practice in front of a full-length mirror. Since your favorite way to step forward is probably the one you do the best, use it for this exercise at first, though you want to eventually practice your takeoff with all of your stepping methods. Begin by moving within your stance: shuffling, bouncing, moving your arms, shoulders and hips. Check to see that your face shows no expression as you move about, especially when you explode forward. Don't bob your eyebrows, bug your eyes or inhale sharply.

With a backfist and forward-foot lunge, it looks like this. Shuffle, bob, weave, fake, *bam!* Your backfist explodes, followed a split second later by your lunge step that explodes forward like a rocket exploding from its launch pad.

Don't hesitate   The difference between doing this with a live partner and doing it in the mirror is that your mirror image is not going to hit you back (you do know that, don't you?). With a live partner, the possibility of him hitting you might psyche you and cause you to hesitate on your way in. Keep in mind that any hesitation, even a fraction of a second, may result with your eating his fist. But if you train hard in front of the mirror and get to a stage where you are doing everything right, your confidence will be high and it will carry over to when you do it with a live person.

Important

Practice repetitively to ensure that all the right elements are there. Even if you are a veteran fighter, spending mirror time to evaluate your initial takeoff is something you should do often. If this concept is new to you, you should devote many solo workouts to it until you are satisfied that you can move like a living rocket.

DOUBLE TAPPING

Double tapping is a shooting technique where the shooter pulls the trigger twice every time he shoots. It's fast and it delivers two deadly bullets to the target in roughly the same amount of time as just one. Say a man, armed with a knife, charges toward a man armed with a gun (which, by the way, is violating the common sense rule "Never take a knife to a gunfight"). The gunman aims at the man's chest and double taps two rounds. The man with the knife continues to advance and the gunman aims at his stomach and double taps again. Finally the assailant falls. Would single shots have stopped the threat? Who knows? I know of three separate incidents where people were shot in the heart and continued to fight for several seconds, some were able to run several hundred yards before they died. Double tapping takes virtually no extra effort, but it dramatically increases the likelihood that the threat will be stopped.

Double tapping your karate technique works in the street, in competition and it's an outstanding way to train to build speed and power. You can double tap most kicks and most of your hand techniques (though some work better than others) and do so with incredible speed. Let's examine how you can do it using your reverse punch.

After you have warmed up your shoulder (don't skip the warm-up because double tapping is fairly strenuous on your muscles and joints), assume your fighting stance, left leg forward. Scoot your left foot out into a forward stance and execute your reverse punch as you normally do. Snap your arm back, and immediately punch again. You can retract it only half way back after the first punch or you can retract it all the way. Although punching from the half-way-back position is not as powerful as when punching from a fully retracted position, it's much faster. Practice both.

Important

A common error when double tapping is to not hit as hard with the second technique as with the first. Be conscious of this and ensure that both blows are landing with all your power. You can hit the same target twice or hit a different target with the second rep. For example, you can drive both reverse punches into the assailant's throat, or put one in his throat and the other into his solar plexus. If great speed is needed, pop two reverses as fast as you can. But if the first blow weakens the attacker and you have an extra second, load up that second punch and drive it in as hard as you are able. Try double tapping with other hand techniques, such as your backfist, jab and roundhouse punch.

Mixing Techniques

Once you feel comfortable using the same technique twice, experiment with mixing two different techniques with the same hand. For example, throw a right reverse punch followed by a right roundhouse punch. Or snap out a lead jab, followed with a lead hook. Combine any techniques you want as long as they flow smoothly into each other. Imagine that the attacker has his guard up and you have to work around it to hit his body.

In the mirror: Each combination - 2 sets, 10 reps -- each arm
On the heavy bag: Each combination - 2 sets, 10 reps -- each arm

BROKEN RHYTHM

This principle has been around for a long time and has been made popular by tournament fighters. It's popular because it works and when done correctly, it works like a charm. It even works for joke tellers: "On the first day, the farmer's daughter meets a traveling salesman and ... The next day, the farmer's daughter meets another traveling salesman and ... On the third day, the farmer's daughter meets one more traveling salesman and *kaboom*" (the punch line). An expectation and a sort of rhythm are established with the first two parts and then it's broken on the third. It works with jokes and it works with karate. This is because we consciously or unconsciously look for patterns and rhythms in nature, and when they are broken, the incongruity makes us laugh if it's a joke and gets us punched when it's a karate technique. Bruce Lee said that an erratic fighter was one of the toughest opponents to deal with.

Although you need to practice broken rhythm techniques against a live opponent to see how he responds to the set up, you can practice them by yourself to develop smoothness and to ingrain the idea into your mind. This ingraining process is important, because often a fighter won't try new ideas against a live opponent who can take advantage of his unpolished moves. If this is you, use your time when training alone to polish your techniques and make them part of your repertoire. Let's take a look at four ways to apply broken rhythm. Practice these in front of a mirror and strive to make them appear believable to an opponent.

Partners

Body Fake

The first method is to use only your body to set up your opponent. Stand before a mirror in your fighting stance, left leg forward. Lower your body, as if you were going to slip in a left hook to your opponent's ribs, and step to the left with your lead foot about 12 inches. Check your image to ensure that you really look as if you are going to sneak a hook. Hesitate there for a second and then slide your left foot back a few inches and hesitate for another second. Again step off to the left about 12 inches with your lead foot, crouch and again look as if you are going to ram in a lead left to the ribs. Scoot your lead foot back and slightly extend your right hand. It's this extended hand that breaks the rhythm of your stepping pattern. When he reaches for it, or at least looks at it and wonders what it's doing, take advantage of his confusion by lunging forward with your right foot and driving your left reverse punch into his middle.

2 sets, 15 reps – both sides

Partial Techniques

This time you establish a rhythm using partial punches or kicks. Try it with your backfist. Stand before the mirror in your fighting stance, left leg forward. Snap a partial backfist, about ½ to 3/4 of the way out, and then dance away. Move forward again and snap out another partial backfist. In just two reps, you have established a rhythm, but now it's time to break it. Move forward a third time and throw out another partial backfist, but extend this one nearly all the way out. Since you have established a pattern in your opponent's mind, make this backfist a tad high to draw his attention upward. As he goes to block it, drive your reverse punch into his ribs. Try not to laugh too hard at him.

2 sets, 15 reps – both sides

Erratic Speed and Footwork

For our purposes here, being erratic is being without rhythm. I suppose it could be argued that there is rhythm within erraticness, but thinking about that just confuses me. Instead, let's move on and look at an example of using erraticness to confuse your opponent.

Erratic speed　Face your imaginary opponent, and on the command of the imaginary referee, explode at him with a flurry of hard and fast punches and kicks. Back off for a moment, dance around for a couple seconds, and then resume sparring but with less intensity. Go for about 20 seconds, and then explode into another all-out series of kicks and punches. Do that for about five seconds, and then switch back to moderate speed again. Can you see how this can confuse your opponent? While he is saying "What the –" you are having a ball scoring on him.

Shadow sparring: 5 minutes

Erratic Footwork

Another way to confuse your opponent as you spar is to use stop-and-go footwork. Dance in and out of range and dance from right to left. Then stop. Pose in your fighting stance for about five seconds and then start dancing again. After a couple times of this, your opponent becomes befuddled. It's at that moment that you explode forward with a fast attack.

Disrupting your Opponent's Rhythm

Workout Tip

Tournaments should be a place of camaraderie, sportsmanship and healthy competition. That said, here is a little way you can cheat. Let's say you are fighting a guy who is having a great tournament day. He has a winning rhythm going that has him ahead on points, and there is only seconds left on the clock. You need to break his rhythm, but how?

Whoops! Your belt came untied; you need to call time out to tie it. Whoops! Your mouthpiece fell out and when you go to pick it up, you accidentally kick it out of the ring. Whoops! His last point hurt you a little and you need a moment to get your breath back.

A "whoops" buys you a moment to get yourself together and it disrupts your hot opponent's rhythm and winning momentum. Don't misunderstand: I'm not suggesting that you cheat. I'm just a reporter reporting what some fighters do. :-)

"Go Nuts"

Although the first system in which I trained way back in 1965 was a traditional one, my instructor was anything but traditional. He didn't use Asian terminology and he didn't bog us down in ritual. He didn't waste time and he didn't waste words. When we worked on combination attacks, he would simply say "Okay, go nuts" and with those two words, we would attack each other as if we had gone totally mad. And that is what I am suggesting you do in this drill, but with control and finesse.

Why you need combinations   Before we get to the actual drill, ponder this: Fights are seldom won with a single blow. Of the countless fights I have witnessed over the years as a cop, it still amazes me how much the human body can tolerate, especially when drugs, alcohol, rage or mental illness is involved. I've seen people shot in the face and heart with a firearm, struck in the head with a hammer, stabbed multiple times and even hit by a car, but still they fought like animals. Yes, they hurt later, or died later, but minutes after their traumatic injury, they were still in there fighting. So, you have to ask yourself this: Is my punch more powerful than a bullet in the face or the bumper of a speeding car? If not, consider hitting multiple times.

Stand in front of a mirror or a heavy bag and throw a two-count combination as a warm up. Do about 10 reps and then add another technique. Do 10 reps of the three-count combination and then add a fourth technique. Continue in this fashion until you are doing a 10-count combination. You can do the same techniques in the same order each time, or you can do whatever techniques you want as long as they flow nicely. I think it's best to just let the techniques happen and not get into a set pattern. But you do it the way that you want.

Strive for efficiency. See if you can get two or three techniques out of each motion. For example, throw a reverse punch, fold your arm and strike with your elbow and then claw with the same hand as you retract your arm.

Training Tip

Hit hard with each blow, especially if you are hitting the mass of your opponent's body. The tendency when throwing multiples is for the blows to weaken as you near the end of your combination. Be cognizant of this and don't let it happen. If you cannot hit hard because of your angle or closeness to the target, then hit a vulnerable target. In the reverse punch/elbow/claw technique just described, your hand is not in a strong position to strike after you have thrown the second technique, the elbow. Therefore, a claw to the face should follow the elbow since power is not necessary to that target.

Strive for speed. Unlike your training partner, a competitor or an assailant isn't going to stand there holding his punch extended while you go nuts on his body. It's imperative, therefore, that you explode your techniques. When using efficiency, you should be able to get all 10 blows in within two seconds.

In the air: 9 sets, 10 reps per set. Begin with a two-count combination and add one technique per set until you are doing 10 reps

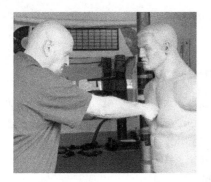

Here is an example of getting three techniques out of one thrust and return. Execute a reverse punch, fold your arm into an elbow smash and then execute a claw as your arm returns to the on-guard position.

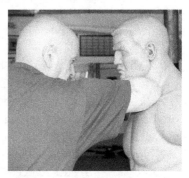

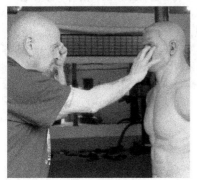

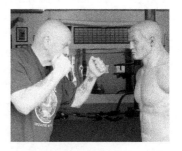

On the bag: 9 sets, 10 reps per set. Begin with a two-count combination and add one technique per set until you are doing 10 reps

TRAIN YOUR OTHER SIDE

When you spar, you probably favor one side more than the other. Right-handed fighters usually emphasize their left side forward, though there are some styles that lead with their strong side, which is usually the right. Whatever your style, you no doubt have one side that you like more than the other. While that is okay, it's important that you never refer to the side you do not like as your "weak side." It may seem like a minor point, but it's important to always keep negativity out of your mind.

All my students are right-handed, and although we give equal time to both sides during our exercises and drills, they still emphasize their left side forward when sparring. Their techniques look fine on their other side and they can hit the bag hard from it. Still, many of them complain that their techniques on that side "feel weird."

I've been training since 1965, and techniques thrown with my ride-side-forward stance still feel differently than when they are thrown with my left side forward, and they probably always will. But no matter how slightly different they feel, my training, classroom and solo training, has provided me with self knowledge as to what I do well and not so well from that side, and from the other side, for that matter. Here are some things you can do to help yourself gain insight into your strengths and limitations on your so-called other side.

Double-up on It

If you have a weakness or self-doubt about your abilities, you should train extra hard until the problem goes away or until you have improved to where you are satisfied. One way to train extra hard on your other side is to double the number of reps you do there. For example when doing a set of 10 reverse punches with your right arm, switch stances and do 20 with your left. If you do 10 right roundhouse kicks, do 20 with your left leg. The idea is to work until you feel comfortable and confident delivering the technique from that other side.

Equally as important, is to develop a *feel* for your other side. Yes, you can execute a right backfist and a right side kick, but it's important that you also thoroughly understand how the techniques feel to all the involved muscles and joints as they extend and return. With this understanding, you are better able to coordinate your muscles and mind to work together.

You won't develop this feel on your other side if you always throw techniques from your favorite side.

HIT HIM WHEN HE IS DOWN

Important

When I played and fought on the school grounds as a child, long before I knew there was such a thing as the martial arts, kicking in a fight was considered unfair, or even worse, it was considered "fighting like a girl." Looking back on it now, I can see that those fighters using their feet were actually years ahead of their time. Even years later in the mid-1960s when karate was quickly becoming a household word, the uninformed would ask, "Karate? Isn't that where you kick with your feet? Isn't that unfair?"

This belief eventually died as the martial arts became more mainstream, but then another misunderstanding took its place, one unfortunately shared by too many martial artists: Never kick or punch a guy when he is down. Fortunately, that belief too has mellowed with time, but there are still fighters who will not do it. This may be because of a school rule where the fighters train, or because of the fighters' belief of what they consider fair.

After you take the assailant down, knock the wind out of him with a hard punch to his lower ribs.

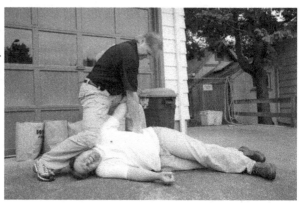

There are tournaments that don't allow kicking or punching a downed fighter. Even in those that do, there are often individual judges who refuse to award points for it. While schools and tournaments nix it for safety and insurance reasons, which is a legitimate concern, it nonetheless teaches fighters a bad habit, one that many street assailants welcome because it gives them a chance to reach for a weapon or at least get back up and have another go at it.

If you have not been training to attack a downed opponent, I encourage you to include finishing blows when you train alone. Here are two ways:

Shadow Sparring

As you move about battling your invisible opponent, imagine foot sweeping him to the ground or driving him down with a series of debilitating blows. Once he is down, prevent him from getting up by hitting him with kicks and punches. See the targets clearly in your mind: Stomp his ankles, knees, thighs, groin, elbows, forearms, upper arms, and face. With your hands, drive punches into his groin, solar plexus and throat.

Shadow sparring: 10 minutes

Self-defense Drills

When you pantomime various self-defense drills when training alone, include a few takedowns with finishing punches and kicks. With some of the takedowns, go down to the floor with your imaginary opponent and roll around on the ground punching and kicking at specific targets that you see clearly in your mind's eye (this is another one of those exercises where you hope no one is looking in the window).

5 reps per self-defense technique

Heavy bag As you practice shadow sparring or the self-defense drills, use a lying heavy bag as your downed opponent. Position yourself so that when you execute the takedown, you are over the bag. Decide which end is the head and which represents the legs and attack it accordingly.

Shadow spar: 10 minutes

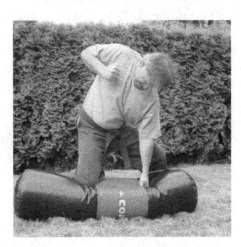

Place a bag on the ground, and as you shadow spar, pantomime dumping your opponent and finishing him off.

The training concept here is to ingrain ground finishing techniques in your mind. But if you never practice them when training alone or training in your school, don't fool yourself by thinking you are automatically going to do it in a real situation. First, the idea has to be in your mind. Training alone is a good place to start the ingraining process.

Caution

Legal tip   In a real self-defense situation, your reason for kicking or punching a downed attacker is because you believe that if you don't he will get up and hurt you. But if it's a situation where he has fallen to the ground and he is indicating that he doesn't want to continue fighting, or it's obvious he is unable to because of injury, there is no self-defense reason for you to kick and punch him further. Either use a restraint hold until help arrives, or run for help and call the police.

But if you do hit him after he has indicated he doesn't want to continue, you could find yourself in trouble with the law.

HIT YOURSELF DRILL

If you don't want to be hauled off in a straight jacket, don't do this drill in a crowded park or in an aisle at the grocery store. It's safer to do it in the privacy of your own training area and to turn up the music to cloak your grunts. The Hit Yourself Drill is a simple and not so fun way to condition yourself to take blows to your body (actually, I can't think of any *fun* way to do it). While there are lots of conditioning drills that involve your training partner kicking and punching you, this one you do alone, which allows you to control the impact and the degree that you increase it.

Boxers and other full contact fighters believe you can physically condition your body to take hard blows, while people in the medical field not only disagree, but talk of its potential danger to vital organs. What I know for sure is that you can *mentally* condition yourself to accept blows so that you do not react to them (except those that debilitate or knock you out). New students react strongly to even the mildest blow, but in about three months, most can take a hard body shot and keep on going. Within half a year, most are able to take hard blows without flinching. If the blow is brought to their attention later, they either shrug it off or don't even remember it happening.

Does this mean they have become impervious to pain? No. But it does mean that they have mentally accepted it as part of their training, just as they have gotten used to sweating, being winded and fatigued (one time, I had a new student who was upset her first night because the training made her sweaty). This simple drill will get you to the acceptance stage faster.

Use any stance you want, but for now let's use the horse stance. If you want to work your legs at the same time, sit low. If you are saving them for another exercise in your workout, sit at any level you want. Begin by striking your thighs. Use the bottoms of both fists to strike each leg, from your knees to your hips and on the inside and outside of your thighs. Reach around and hit the backs of your legs. Now strike your ribs, abdomen, chest and your sides as far around as you can reach.

Do 5 minutes, each training session

USE YOUR HEAD

People on the receiving end of a headbutt, know how nasty it can be.

Imagine that you are a street creep entertaining your three, IQ-deficient buddies by taunting and threatening a man who is waiting for a bus. You jab your finger against his chest and say things about his mother. When you grab his shirt front and pull him toward you to scare him, his head makes a funny move, followed by a sudden, bolt of white pain streaking through your brain as your nose explodes over your face and clothes.

Now you too know how nasty headbutts can be.

First, Strengthen your Neck

You should consistently incorporate neck exercises in your regular conditioning program, such as wrestlers' bridges, weight resistance exercises and exercises using specific neck machines found in many health clubs. Besides helping you develop a powerful headbutt, a strong neck is vitally important to lessen the shock and concussion from head blows and falls. Additionally, a powerful looking neck improves your appearance, making you look strong and less like a pencil-neck victim. Neck exercises are easy to do and for most people the neck responds faster than other muscle groups.

Exercise for the back of the neck: 3 sets, 15 reps
Exercise for the front of the neck: 3 sets, 15 reps

(The sides of the neck are stimulated sufficiently by exercises for the front and back)

To work the muscles at the front of your neck, assume the position shown and, by pushing off the balls of your feet, gently roll your head forwards and back. You can increase the intensity of the exercise by adjusting the position of your feet.

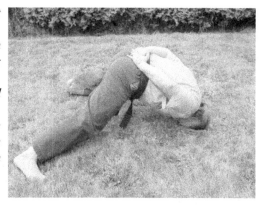

To strengthen the back of your neck, assume the position shown and gently roll your head back and then forward.

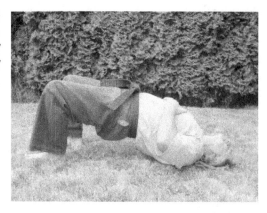

Point of Impact

Strike with the crown of your head, that area where the band of your hat touches. Any other impact point, such as your face or the back of your head near your neck, is going to knock you silly.

Caution

Targets

The primary targets are the attacker's nose, chin, temple and ear. Smashing your forehead into his nose will cause acute pain and immediate and severe tearing of his eyes. A blow to his temple, that area in front of his ear, is excruciatingly painful and may cause unconsciousness. Impact to his ear is painful and may cause disorientation. A blow to his chin may knock him out and break his jaw.

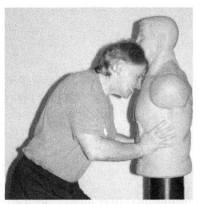

Manakin-type bags are perfect for headbutt practice, but any bag will do. When you are under his head, seize the opportunity to snap your head up into his chin.

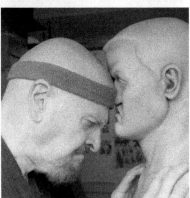

When in a clinch, slam your head (the area covered by the sweatband) into your attacker's nose.

The Body Mechanics of the Headbutt

Important

Many fighters think of headbutting as pulling their head back to chamber, and then whipping it forward into the target. Not only is that a weak way to deliver it, it's potentially dangerous to your neck. Instead, think of the action coming from your lower back while you hold your neck straight and stiff, similar to a short bow.

Front headbutt   Stand before your hanging bag, goofy bag or manikin-type bag. It's important to have a specific target to strike, so if you don't have one with a face, draw one on your heavy bag. Since headbutting is not a long-range technique, begin by snuggling up close to the bag. Keep your neck stiff and press your tongue against the roof of your mouth so as not to bite it. Snap your upper body forward from your waist and smack your head into the bag. Remember to hit with the crown of your head.
2 sets, 10 reps

Side headbutt   Face your bag with your arms around it as if in a clinch and then lean forward and to the side of your bag. Using your waist, snap your upper body toward the target and strike it with the side of your head. Think of it as striking an assailant in the temple or ear.
2 sets, 10 reps – both sides

Rear headbutt   To practice defending against an assailant who has grabbed you from behind in a bear hug, stand with your back to the bag and snap your upper body back, striking the target with the crown portion at the back of your head. You can use the same part of your head to strike the assailant's chin when your head is underneath, such as when grappling or in a clinch. Bring your head up sharply, striking him with the crown of your head. If you don't have a manikin-type bag, a goofy bag works well.
2 sets, 10 reps

Combinations

This is where it gets really interesting, not to mention highly destructive to your assailant. Imagine a real person as you experiment with these on your bag and in the air. Since headbutting is a close range technique, there is little or no footwork involved other than a short shuffle in or to the side.

- Strike with a front headbutt into his nose two times. Imagine his head snapping back on the first one and then as it returns, strike him again.
- Move in at an angle to your left and then snap the right side of your head into his temple. Draw your head and upper body back in one fluid motion and then front headbutt his nose.
- Move in at an angle to your right and snap the side of your head into his. In one, continuous motion, move your head past his face until it's on the other side of his head and then headbutt that side. In other words, first headbutt his left side and then his right side.

The more you practice, the more combinations you discover. Headbutting is a devastating technique that should be in your repertoire.

GETTING UP FROM THE GROUND

No matter what your ground-fighting skill, being down while your assailant is on his feet is not a good place to be. Yes, grappling competitors love the mat and have developed offensive and defensive techniques that turn their opponents into overly-twisted pretzels. But that is on the mat. In the dark, dank street, however, being down means that you are lying on asphalt or cement and, in case you didn't know, asphalt and cement are not your friends. As a police officer who experienced a multitude of fights on the ground, I always, and I do mean always, left little patches, sometimes big patches, of my skin on the flesh-eating street.

Cement burns are the least of your worries when a street assailant looks down at you sprawled out on the ground, the same

Important

way a vulture looks at fresh roadkill. Even worse is when one or more of his buddies are looking at you the same way. Being down when the assailant, or assailants, move in to finish you off, makes you vulnerable to getting hit, stabbed or shot, and it greatly reduces the power of your offensive techniques.

When training alone, practice getting up from the ground quickly and defensively, two critical elements since the vultures are probably going to attack while you are doing it. Consider the following tips to help you get to your feet bruise free.

Continue Fighting as you Stand Up

My mother enjoyed baseball and played it as a teenager. One of the techniques she taught me when fielding ground balls was to bend, catch the ball and without standing up, throw it to the appropriate base. Throwing while bent saves critical time since a fraction of a second can make the difference whether the runner is called out or declared safe. In a real fight, a fraction of a second can also make a difference as to whether you are out or safe. Let's take a look at my mother's technique as it applies to your getting off the floor while the assailant is still in striking range.

Lie down and imagine your assailant moving in to finish you off. Examine ways to punch, kick and block at every stage of your standing up.

- When lying on your back or on your stomach
- As you sit up
- When you are sitting up
- As you get up on one or both knees
- When you are up on one or both knees
- When you are half way to a standing position
- When standing
2 sets, 10 reps – in each stage

Here are two ways to get up suggested by Instructor Steve Golden. To make these methods safer, he advises that no matter how you fall, always keep your head out of the line of fire by twisting your body so that your feet are between you and the threat.

Roll Onto your Side

Say you are on your back or sitting on your rear. Golden says, "In all the jujitsu that I've ever seen, they show how to get up in a very safe manner without using your hands. I don't like that. Here is what I do like. I tell the opponent, 'Okay. You win. I've had enough,' or something of that nature. While saying that, I tuck my feet up to my chest as I sit up, roll slightly on my left side, put my left hand on the ground and push myself up to my feet. Although this looks like I'm putting myself in danger, the position actually lines up my right leg with the opponent in case he attacks. I can kick his closest knee, or if he is reaching downward, I can kick right to his face using my left hand on the ground for support.

"To practice, get on your back, pull your legs up as you roll slightly to your left and place your left hand on the ground for support and to help push you up. Every second repetition, shoot out your right kick as you drop back down. You can use your hand to push yourself closer to the attacker, to make the kick even stronger."

2 sets, 10 reps – both sides

Runner's Position

Say you have landed face down, or you have landed on your back and rolled over onto your stomach. With your arms, push up your upper body as you look back over either shoulder at the threat. Golden says, "Bring your knees up to your chest, and then, in a position that looks like you are getting ready to run away, push yourself up with your arms and stand with either foot first. At any point as you get up, you can mule kick back with your bent, forward leg when the opponent closes the distance."

2 sets, 10 reps

When you are training alone and having an aerobic workout, include 5-10 minutes of simply getting up and down from the floor. It's a real energy drainer and will have you huffing and puffing. It will also begin to ingrain in your mind ways to get up with speed, balance and a ready defense.

SLIPPING

Slipping is a defensive movement that not only keeps you from getting hit, but positions you to throw a solid counter blow. It's an evasive snap of your head and upper body to the left, right or back. Muhammad Ali was a master of slipping, often making his hapless opponents look foolish as they punched the air where his head has been less than a second earlier.

Slipping with Speed

I used to believe that slipping was ineffective because a fast puncher can move his little fist much faster than I can move my big ol' body. By experimenting, however, I discovered that if I could perceive the attack just as it began, my chance of successfully slipping was much greater. But if I waited until the attack was halfway to me before I tried to slip it, I got bopped in the noggin.

It's also helpful to snap your hand up to swat the blow aside in conjunction with the slip. This way you have two things going for you: You move your body out of the line of trajectory, and you snap out a block in case your body is having an especially slow day. With your blocking hand up, you are in a good position to sneak in a fast counter. Say you slip to the left and snap your right hand up to swat aside his jab. As easy as pie, you can drive in a right palm strike to his nose and, just for laughs, a left roundhouse into his ribs. Be careful not to always move in the same direction with a real opponent, since a savvy one will quickly figure out your pattern.

Training Tip

When pulling your head back to avoid a punch, don't lean so far that it throws you off balance. Muhammad Ali was one of the few who could successfully lean way back, but that was because his waist was like a rubber band.

*Your assailant launches a left jab at you. Evade it with a quick slip to
your right and counter with a right punch.*

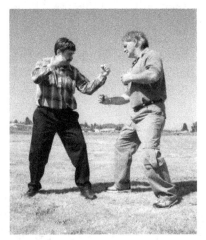 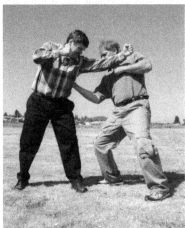

Solo slipping   Here are a couple ways you can practice
slipping when training alone. Pay attention to your speed (are you
able to move faster in one direction than the other?) and the position of your hands, so you can get off quick counters.

Mirror time: Square off against that ugly opponent in the
mirror. Make sure your hands are up and begin moving around as if
sparring your image. As you do so, snap your head and upper body
to the left and then to the right. Next time, quickly lean your head
and body back a little. Important: Don't overextend in any direction
and never give up your balance. Once you feel comfortable that your
form is good, pick up the speed.

Important

You can include this exercise when training alone, or if you
lift weights, do it for one minute between sets.

Shadow sparring: 2, 60-second rounds

Double-end bag: This is especially effective because if you
don't slip correctly, you get a mouth full of vinyl. Punch the bag and
slip to the right or left when it pops back. Let it go back out and
then hit it on its return. This time when it returns, slip to the left or

right as you snap up a backhand block and shoot out a punch to the air with the same hand as if you were hitting your opponent's body.

Keep in mind that the harder you hit it, the faster it comes back. So if you are just learning to slip, hit it easy at first and then progressively hit harder as you improve.

5 sets, 60-second rounds

Heavy bag: The heavy bag isn't as effective as is the double-end bag for slipping practice, but if it's on a fast swivel it can come back fairly hard and knock you off balance when you are day dreaming. Slip to avoid it and then punch, kick or push it. Consider using the heavy bag to work on moving your entire body out of the way and use the double-end bag to practice slipping your head and upper body.

2 sets, 60-second rounds

Work the clock   Assume your fighting stance on your taped asterisk and begin shadow sparring. Step off to 9 o'clock and slip your head to the left as if evading a punch. Counter with a right roundhouse kick. Move back and face 12 o'clock and then duck quickly to the right toward 3 o'clock to avoid his jab. Counter with a backfist to his groin and with additional punches as you straighten back up. Continue to work the clock, slipping and countering with strong counters. Use vivid imagery so that you are aware of your imaginary opponent's position when you move away from his attack. Whenever you slip in the direction of his free hand, check it with your hand as you deliver a sharp counter.

5 set, 60-second rounds

NATURAL STANCE

As the name implies, natural stance is your natural way of standing. Your legs are not spread and your hands are not in an on-guard position. It's how you stand when you are in line at the grocery store. While many fighters don't think of it as a combat stance, it's the position in which most real fights occur. Real fighting often erupts so fast that you don't get a chance to drop into your sparring stance and, even if you could, you may not want to since it would give away your element of surprise. To make your natural stance a fighting stance, you have to first *think* of it as a fighting stance and then *train* with it as such. Once you have it ingrained in your mind, you will always be combat ready.

Stand before a mirror in your natural stance. Launch your basic reverse punch with a forward step, and then return to your natural stance. For your next rep, step backward and punch. On each punch, examine how to use your body mechanics to make the punch as strong as you are able while minimizing telegraphing. What other hand techniques are easy to do from your natural stance? Which ones are awkward and which ones require too much telegraphing? Which kicks are fast and efficient from your natural stance? Which ones are not? How do you best use your body to make your kick as powerful as possible? How do your blocks work in your natural stance? Can you do them without taking a step back?

Find the answer to these questions when training alone so that you know what you can and cannot use when that street thug steps out of the alley directly into your path. Knowledge is power.

2 sets, 10 reps of each technique you choose – both sides

BAG WORK: NO GLOVES OR FOOT PROTECTION

For hand and wrist safety, it's a good idea to wear gloves when pounding the heavy bag. Boxers and Muay Thai fighters wrap their hands for even more protection before they slip on the gloves. That said, I want to encourage you to pound the bag occasionally without hand protection to get a feel for what it's like hitting with your bare hands. You are not going to be wearing gloves out in the street, so hitting someone for the first time without hand protection may distract you for a moment, and a moment of distraction in a real fight can be disastrous.

Caution

If you have tender, little hands (and you know who you are without my mentioning names here), don't hit the bag as hard as you do when wearing gloves. You can still experience the feel without pounding away with all your might and removing patches of skin. The same is true with kicks. The tops of my feet are extremely tender (I'm bearing my soul to you), so I have to wear foot protection when I roundhouse kick the heavy bag. Once or twice a month, however, I get naked from my ankles down, and kick with my bare feet, though I don't even come close to doing it as hard as I am able. I kick it with just enough impact to get the experience of hitting without protection.

Bare hand techniques, 5 minutes, once or twice a month
Bare foot techniques, 5 minutes, once or twice a month

DRILL WITH SHOES

If you normally train barefoot or wear protective foam shoes, train occasionally while wearing your street shoes. Just as hitting the heavy bag without hand or foot protection educates you as to the different feel, wearing street shoes also provides you with important information as to any adjustments you have to make in your footwork and kicks. For example, if you wear shoes with rough soles, you are going to discover that your foot doesn't rotate the same way your bare foot does. In fact, it may not rotate at all, which can cause knee injuries when your leg begins to rotate but your foot sticks to the floor due to your shoe's super traction. On the flip side, some dress shoes have extremely slippery soles, so that when you take that quick side step, you may slide right into the splits. And if you normally can't do the splits, that's going to hurt—a lot.

Training
Tip

What adjustments do you have to make in your footwork while wearing slick soled shoes? Running shoes? Slippers? Sandals? Boots? Does it hurt your knee to kick hard while wearing heavy boots? Can you front kick the heavy bag with the ball of your foot while wearing boots? Is your chamber slower when wearing heavy shoes?

SHOULDER AND HIP RAMMING

Have you considered using your shoulders and hips to ram your opponent when the fight gets close and personal. Why not? Football players use their shoulders to send their rivals hard to the ground and jujitsu fighters use their hips to knock the wind out of their opponents as they execute hip throws. Indeed, your shoulders and hips are powerful weapons that can cause injury and help you escape a clinch or an assailant's hold.

Ramming in a Clinch

Shoulder ram   You can charge across a room and shoulder ram someone, but for now, let's consider using it at close range. Say you are clinching with an attacker and you cannot get off a punch. As you jostle around with him, take advantage of any moment when you sense that one of his hands has a weak grip, and drive your same-side shoulder into whatever you can hit – his arms, chest, abdomen, shoulders, face – using the thrusting power of your legs and upper body. What you do as a follow-up depends on how he reacts to the ram.

There are two methods of shoulder ramming:

Facing-shoulder ram: Face the bag from about 18 inches away. Snap your upper body forward as you simultaneously twist it to the right and hit the target with your left shoulder. The twist adds a tad more impact to the blow as opposed to just bending forward and striking.

2 sets, 10 reps — each shoulder

Side-shoulder ram: Stand sideways to the bag, about 18 inches away. As explosively as you are able, step sideways with your closest foot, dip your upper body and ram your left shoulder into the bag.

2 sets, 10 reps — both shoulders

Hip ram   The hip ram is not as powerful as the shoulder ram, but when it impacts your opponent's lower stomach, groin and upper thigh, it can be quite painful. I have had jujitsu fighters ram their pile-driving hips into me so hard that the hip blow hurt more than the throw that followed. Hip ramming should be considered a close-in fighting technique, unless you can think of a situation where you would run across an open space and hip thrust someone.

When grabbed from behind, arms free or pinned, a powerful thrust backward with your hips can do much to weaken the attacker's grip. I know a guy who can do it so hard that it often sends his opponent sliding on his rear across the floor. It's also effective against a bear hug from the side. Depending on the height difference between you and your opponent, your hip strikes his lower abdomen, groin or upper thighs.

Important

Use the same concept in a clinch as you did with the shoulder ram technique. When you feel a weakness in his grip, ram your same-side hip into him. Do it a couple times if you have the opportunity, and then break free and run or counter with punches and kicks. When the attacker is pushing you all over the place, it's virtually impossible to execute a hip ram. But when there is a pause in the struggle or he pulls you into him, ram your hip into whatever target you can hit. Here are a couple of ways you can do it alone.

When clinching with an opponent, take advantage of any weakness in his grip to slam your hip into his lower abdomen/groin area.

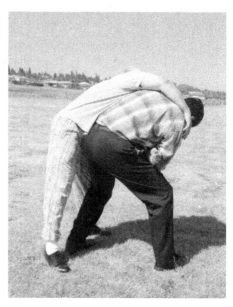

Facing hip rams   Face the bag from about 18 inches away. Step forward with your left leg, turn your hip toward the bag, and ram it.

2 sets, 10 reps — both sides

Side-hip rams   Stand sideways to the bag, nearly touching it. Simultaneously, twist on the ball of your closest foot as you snap your hip into the bag.

2 sets, 10 reps — both sides

You have to experiment with your body angling and foot placement to determine where your power lies. I encourage you to experiment with shoulder and hip rams because they may be the one thing that gets you out of a bad situation.

THE GOOD OLD PUSH

Sometimes karate fighters get so caught up in the fancy-smancy techniques that they don't consider the simple ones, such as the good ol' push. Have you ever seen a sumo wrestler push his opponent? Those mountains of flesh (apologies to any sumo wrestlers who might be reading this) practice for hours shoving each other and slamming their palms so hard against huge posts buried in the ground that the thumping sound can be heard blocks away. If you weighed 160 pounds and got pushed by one of these guys, you would starve to death before you stopped rolling down the sidewalk. Unless you weigh 500 pounds and slam tree trunks for a workout, let me be the one to break this to you: You will never possess a shove as powerful as a sumo wrestler's. Nonetheless, you can still develop a powerful one.

Here is an effective method of pushing that you can easily practice by yourself.

Upward Tai Chi Push

I learned this method of pushing while studying tai chi, the so-called "gentle art." By the way, I learned quickly not to write off tai chi just because the practitioners move slowly; they have some sneaky and incredibly painful moves. Consider their upward push.

As you face an opponent, drop your open palms to the level of your belt and then thrust them slightly upward as you step forward. Slam your palms just below his rib cage on both sides, and push forcefully in an upward, 45-degree direction. When executed at combat speed, this push causes a tremendous shock to the recipient's rib cage, or as my instructor used to say, it "ruptures his chassis." Even a mild push there will shock the recipient.

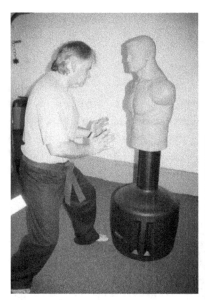

As you face the bag, thrust both palms forward and upward at about a 45-degree angle, striking it in the area of the lower ribs.

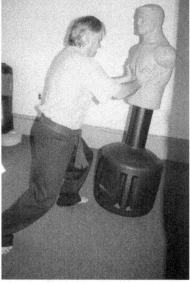

Pushing upward on the heavy bag   Stand in front of a heavy bag in your natural stance or fighting stance. Drop your hands to your hips on a level with your belt and thrust your palms out as you lunge toward the bag. Your palms should take off a fraction of a second before your lead foot lunges. Slam your palms where you would imagine an average-sized person's ribs to be, and push upward at a 45-degree angle. If your angle is correct, the bag should lift upward slightly and wobble.

2 sets, 10 reps

Here are three exercises to develop power in your tai chi push:

Bench press   A policeman friend, who has never studied the martial arts, began working extra hard on his bench press. He made remarkable progress in a year, developing muscle mass and increasing the poundage on the bar more than he ever imagined. One night, a suspect pushed him against a wall and drew his fist back, the kind of fist that has "Six months in the hospital" written across the knuckles. Reflexively, my friend slammed his palms against the guy's chest and gave a mighty push, just as he did thrice weekly with a 375-pound barbell. The suspect, his arms flailing, hurtled backwards through tables and chairs, knocking several over along the way. When his back hit the edge of the bar, he belched out a loud "Oooomff!" before sliding slowly to the floor, where he sat struggling for air. My friend says he owes it all to those bench presses.

The bench press is probably the best supplemental exercise for developing power in the push. I highly recommend you do them a couple times a week and strive to build strength.

Workout Tip

4-6 sets, 8 to 10 reps

Straight-in push on the bag   The straight-in push is an exercise that works your pushing muscles from a slightly different angle than the tai chi push. You can also use this push as a fighting technique. For example, say there is an opening in the struggle but you don't have time to drop your body and push upward. Seize the moment and push straight in. It does not have the same shock effect as the upward push, but it still gets the assailant off of you.

Stand in front of a motionless bag (the heavier the better) and step forward with either leg and double palm it. Rotate your hand so that your fingers are pointing out to each side at about a 45-degree angle. Slam straight into the bag using the muscles of your arms, chest and shoulders.

3 sets, 10 reps

Medicine ball thrust   Lie on your back and hold a medicine ball on your chest. With explosive power, thrust the ball straight up as high as you can make it go. Catch it on its way down, and allow it to sink back to your chest where, without hesitation, you thrust it straight back up again. Each set is done nonstop.

3 sets, 10 reps

Tai-Yang Lung Tao push

I learned this push from Instructor Kenneth Smith. It's a marvelous technique that, like many others that are based on leverage, works so easily that it appears you have mystical power. Hey, let people believe what they want about you.

Here is what Kenneth Smith said when I asked about his push. "I wish it were my technique, but I have to give credit to Fong Su-Yi, creator of Tai-Yang Lung Tao. When either of the following exercises are translated into practice with a living partner, you will simply not believe how effortless it feels to control the movements of an attacker. You will be absolutely astounded by your ability to topple a much larger and stronger assailant." Here is how it works.

Say the attacker comes at you with a shoulder-high push. Smith says: "Place the palms of your hands on either side of his body, near or below his lower ribs. Keep your elbows down at your sides and allow the forward pressure of his attack to slightly compress your weight into the ground through your rear leg. Now, before he can tip you over, shift your whole body along a sweeping arc, upward and back down onto your forward foot. This should, if performed properly, make you feel like a coiled spring. The elastic quality of your body's muscle tissues will allow you to effortlessly expand outward and downward at about a 45-degree angle, uprooting your opponent

Partners

and propelling him backward at an alarming rate. His weight will drop onto his rear foot, making his front one 'empty' and toppling him. You do not, however, have to shove him away. Instead, your concentration should be upon the upward and downward circle and the shift of your body weight, which will redirect the force of his attack and send him sailing."

Smith suggests the following two exercises to develop the feel of the push.

Kitchen chair push   "Stand in front of a kitchen chair, with the seat facing you. The back of a standard chair will be about as high as an opponent's waist. By pushing downward at a 45-degree angle against the back of the chair, you can easily tip it over. You can even put some weight on the chair to increase its resistance, but be careful of the chair legs as they rise up off the floor. They are like the legs of an opponent as he falls over backwards, so you don't want to get caught by them and thrown to the ground yourself.

"Practicing with a chair is far more awkward than practicing with a human partner, but, it serves its purpose. If you can control the angle and energy of a weighted chair with style and grace, then a human opponent will seem like magic. Your assailant will seem to throw himself to the floor, with little or no effort on your behalf."

10 minutes, or do until smooth

Beach ball push   Smith offers another exercise to strengthen the Tai-Yang Lung Tao push. "Another practice method is to stand in waist-deep water in a swimming pool (I personally prefer the natural feel of a lake or the ocean) and push a beach ball under. You will have to maintain contact with it at all times, or it will pop away, and you must push at the proper angle. If you push at less than 45 degrees, the ball will simply roll out of your grasp; if you push it at more than 45, it will require a lot of energy to submerge it and even more to control it. This is a great exercise to develop the sensitivity needed to control the path of your attacker's energy, but it does not give you the feel of toppling an actual human opponent."

10 minutes or do until smooth

EYES CLOSED

Important

This exercise will make you aware of all the little things that occur to your body in general and your muscles in particular when you execute a technique. When you cannot see, you can feel the essence of a technique to a greater degree. You can feel how your legs and feet move, how your upper body turns, leans or tilts, how your shoulders rotate, how your arms extend and how your head turns. You will realize quickly how important your sight is to maintaining your balance.

Experiment with the following basics with your eyes closed. You will find that some techniques are not a problem, while others (the turning back kick comes to mind), may trip you and send you toppling out an opened window. At first, do them without stepping, and then when you feel you are ready, experiment with various forms of footwork.

Reverse Punch, 2 sets, 10 reps — both sides
Backfist, 2 sets, 10 reps — both sides
Lead jab, reverse punch, and elbow, 2 sets, 10 reps — both sides
Front kick, 2 sets, 10 reps — both sides
Side kick, 2 sets, 10 reps — both sides
Roundhouse kick, 2 sets, 10 reps — both sides
Turning back kick (close the window) 2 sets, 10 reps — both sides

How to Strengthen your Balance

Have you noticed that there are some days when your balance does not make it to class with you? You throw a kick at the heavy bag or charge against your opponent with a punch, and suddenly you are stumbling and flailing your arms in a desperate struggle to stay upright. We all have those days from time to time; expect them and don't worry about them. But if you consistently lose your balance, you need to work on it.

I have noticed that a person's balance can "get out of shape." So, about every third month, I have my students stand in place and raise their legs out to their sides, to their front and around behind them without touching them to the floor. If they wave their arms and hop around the room to keep from falling, they know that they need to spend time "strengthening" their balance. The good news is that it's not hard to do, and it only takes a few workouts to get it back, sometimes as few as two.

If you are just starting out in the martial arts and your balance is poor, know that it will get better as you continue studying. Also, know that you can speed up your progress by spending a few minutes with the following exercises. If you are a veteran student, and your balance has become poor, add these exercises to your workout to regain your balance in just a few days.

Eyes closed 1   Stand normally and close your eyes. Now, slowly extend your right leg into a front kick. Do you notice how all your little muscles and some big ones are making lots of adjustments to keep you from falling? Those are the ones you are conditioning with this simple exercise. Keep your arms in your on-guard position and resist waving them around.

30 seconds, each leg for a total of 5 minutes

Eyes closed 2   Stand normally with your eyes closed and lift your right knee until your thigh is parallel to the floor. Keep your leg bent and your arms in your on-guard position as you lean your body to the right, left, back and forward.

30 seconds, each leg for a total of 5 minutes

Eyes open 1   Assume your fighting stance, eyes open, arms in your on-guard position and execute a slow front kick. Retract it to your chamber and then execute a slow side kick. Retract and execute a slow roundhouse kick and retract and execute a back kick. Do all four kicks and any others you want to include with the same leg, slowly and without returning your foot to the floor. Fight the urge to wave your arms around for balance.

1 set, 15 reps – both legs

Eyes open 2   This might seem silly, but it's a good way to get a little balance practice in during the day. When you scan the newspaper in the morning before taking off to school or work, do it standing on one leg. You can do it with your raised foot dangling in the air or you can rest it against the knee of your support leg. If you have a private office at work, read those reports with one leg up. When you are in your room reading that book for history class, do it on one leg.

30 seconds each leg – alternate legs for 5 minutes

Incense burner   Let's flip the calender back, oh, say about 400 years. The place: a Shaolin Temple in China where you are being tested as to your worthiness to train with the temple master. You have to lift a large iron incense burner with both hands and hold it in front of you as you support the bottom of it with one of your bent legs. The burner is scalding hot and the engraved dragons on each side burn a scar into your forearms.

Okay, back to the present. Take away the burner and you are left with the pose, arms spread and rounded as if holding that big pot, your finger tips touching. Bend your support leg and lift your other foot as high up your support leg as you are able (imagine that incense burner resting on the big-toe side of it). Keep your back straight, shoulders down, and breath deeply to maintain a state of relaxation. Keep your eyes open and focus on a spot across the room.

Strive for three minutes on each leg the first time and progress over your solo workouts until you are standing for 20-30 minutes, switching from one leg to the other

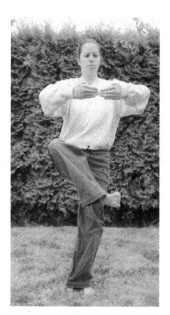

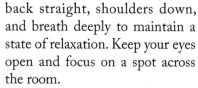

Circle your arms and touch your fingertips, bend your support leg slightly and raise your other leg as pictured. Do three minutes on each leg, and alternate them for 20-30 minutes.

as you tire. If you would rather use your training time to punch and kick, do the incense burner exercise while watching television. It doesn't require great concentration, and the television program will distract you from the discomfort in your muscles. However, if you do want to work on your concentration, leave the television off and assume the position. Focus on a single spot on the wall and breath deeply and rhythmically, while maintaining total relaxation.

1 set, 3–30 minutes – alternating legs every 2 to 3 minutes

EYE DRILLS

Here are several exercises you can do to improve your ability to see the target you are hitting and any other action that is happening. For example, while you drive your fist into your opponent's solar plexus, he launches a front snap kick to your groin. You don't see his kick, however, because you are too focused on the spot that you are hitting. This is called tunnel vision, because it's as if you are looking at your opponent through a toilet paper tube. Your intention to hit your opponent is so great that you see only what is in that small circle. Stress in a real fight or in competition can cause tunnel vision, too. The following exercise can help you control this dangerous phenomenon.

Stalking a busy wall   Try to find a peg board, a large one with thousands of holes or a wall that has a multitude of marks, such as paint splatters or wallpaper with thousands of small designs on it. The busier the better. Find a spot near the middle and focus on it. Now, begin to move about as if you were sparring with someone. Don't throw techniques, but rather use whatever footwork you want to shuffle to the right about 10 feet, to the left about 10 feet, back about 10 feet and then forward about 10 feet. As you move, maintain a total, visual focus on that spot, while still being aware of all the other spots in your peripheral vision.

This might make your eyes spin like those of a cartoon character who has been bopped in the head with a mallet, but keep at it. It's a good exercise to develop your ability to see subtleties in your opponent's movements.

3, 1- minute rounds

Hitting toward a busy wall   Stand in your fighting stance before that marked wall and find a spot on which to focus. Look only at that one spot but be aware of all the others in your peripheral vision, such as how far out they spread and any irregularities in the wall pattern. Stay in place and throw a backfist at the spot. See it, hit it, all the while maintaining awareness of the rest of the wall. This helps you develop the ability to see a small opening in your opponent's defense, while still being aware of the rest of him.

1 set, 10 reps — both sides

Shadow sparring a busy wall   Once again you find yourself before that deadly wall. Pick a spot and begin shuffling around as you do when stalking an opponent. Maintain eye contact with the spot and throw, say, a side kick at it, then a jab, followed by a front kick/reverse punch combination. Bob, weave, block, kick and punch, never taking your eyes from that spot and always being aware of all the other spots in your peripheral vision.

3, 1— minute rounds

Fast focus drill   I learned this drill many years ago from one of my arnis teachers, Leonard Trigg, who learned it while studying stick and knife fighting in the Philippines. It's a no-sweat exercise that you can do even in a chair, though in the beginning you should practice in your fighting stance. Its purpose is to increase your ability to turn in any direction and focus immediately on an approaching threat. With practice, you will be able to see and recognize even the smallest detail.

Here is why this is important. Say you hear or sense something at your side. You turn and see someone, who for the first second or two is not vividly clear. As he comes into focus, you see that it's a man. He is moving toward you. He is lifting his arm. He is gripping a knife.

Although this visual assessment happened quickly, it might not be quick enough. Reread that last paragraph. See how it took five sentences to describe the man and what he is doing? With training, however, you can improve your perception speed so that what you perceive can be described in one fast sentence: *You turn and see a man attacking you with a knife.* Fast perception is especially important if the man has just sharpened that knife. Here is the drill.

Turn and focus drill   First, select one focus point on each of the four walls that surround you. The spot might be a crack, a nail or a design on grandma's scarf in a photograph. It doesn't matter what it is as long as it's small and forces you to focus hard. Do not stand in the center of the room because that will make the focus points the same distance away on all four walls. For the drill to be more beneficial, stand closer to one wall, or to two walls, such as the one on the right and the one directly behind you.

Assume your fighting stance. Turn quickly to your left and focus on your preselected spot on that wall. Bring it into clear focus as quickly as you can and then resume your initial position facing forward. Snap your head to the right and focus on the next small spot. This one might be within an arm's reach or it might be 20 feet away, depending on where you are standing. Resume your initial position and then turn 180 degrees to focus on a spot on the back wall. Return to your initial position and look at the floor in front of your feet. Look up quickly and focus on whatever spot you have selected to your front.

Practice repetitiously looking to your left, right, rear and front. When you feel you are getting good at it, change the focus spot and the distances each time you look. Sometimes look 20 feet away and high, other times look five feet away and low. Keep in mind that the idea is to look fast and bring the spot into focus fast.

10 minutes

EYES AS A TARGET

If an assailant cannot see you, his ability to continue his attack as well as his desire to do so, is drastically reduced. I can't imagine anyone being able to tolerate a finger in their eye, but there is always that possibility; I've been surprised before what people can tolerate. Thus far, however, it's been my experience that even the biggest guy dances around in agony when he gets a gnat in one of his eyes. Imagine how he would dance if you crammed all five of your fingers in them.

The real beauty of using eye techniques ("beauty" may not be the right word) is that you do not need power to cause an effect,

Use a manakin-type bag to develop accuracy for eye techniques.

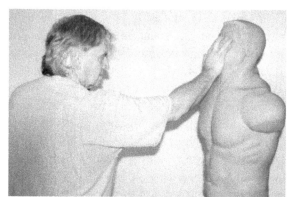

you do not have to be in a particular stance and, in many situations, you do not need to be fast. All you need is a clear path to get your boney fingers into his oh-so-sensitive baby blues.

Steve Perry, a veteran martial artist, professional sci-fi writer and former certified physician's assistant, describes the trauma that can occur when the eyes are attacked. Keep in mind that these are only general possibilities and if you are interested in more detail, you should seek out information from a doctor or in medical literature. I asked Steve for a layman's explanation as to what happens when the eyes are raked and when they are gouged.

"Rakes," he said, "assuming they aren't too deep, usually involve scratching the cornea or the conjunctiva. Deeper rakes might involve the iris and pupil, of course, but just for the sake of explanation, let's make the rake a superficial one to the cornea. It's painful, but generally not dangerous to one's vision. If it isn't too bad, the recipient can put some drops in the affected eye, put a patch on it, and it will get well in a two or three days. This tissue heals very quickly. If the rake went into the eye deeply, the fingers could snag the iris or cornea, even the lens, and that would be very damaging."

For our purposes here, a gouge occurs when a finger(s) is thrust straight into the eye. Steve said: "Gouges can do all kinds of trauma, depending on how hard the impact is, the angle, and the recipient's physiology. A thumb in the eye is very painful, and can cause hemorrhage, either superficially or into the anterior chamber, lacerations to the iris, and the lens and retina can be knocked out of place. A really hard gouge can displace the entire globe, or even tear through it to the vitreous, causing that to leak. It's possible to blow out an orbital-floor with impact to the socket or the eye itself. This is a medical emergency because a blown-out socket can lead to loss of the eye if untreated."

Can eye rakes and gouges cause blindness? Perry says: "It depends on the amount of trauma. If the vitreous humor leaks out, yes. Major mechanical damage to the eye structures, major bleeding and increases in ocular pressure can also result in blindness. Pulling an eye from the socket and damaging the optic nerve would likely do it. There are cases of entire globes coming out whole, being carefully replaced by doctors, and the recovery was total, but I wouldn't bet on that. Once the eye is dangling on your cheek, chances are it won't be seeing things again."

Staying out of the slammer: While you always need to be justified to use force against another person, poking a person in the eyes carries with a it negative connotation to most people, especially judges and juries. If your self-defense situation ever goes to court, the typical jury is going to squirm in discomfort when the assailant's attorney tells them how you, you big brute, gouged his helpless client's eyes in a sadistic attempt to blind him so that he could never see his children again.

Caution

My point is this: Your self-defense situation should warrant the severe degree of force that is eye gouging and eye raking. Some may argue that it's no more serious than kicking someone in the groin or breaking their elbow, but there is a connotation about eye techniques that make people extremely uncomfortable. And if those people are sitting in judgement of you—that is not a good thing.

Okay. That said, here are several eye poking drills you can practice alone.

Block and Gouge

Stand in your fighting stance, left leg forward. With your left palm, swat your imaginary assailant's reverse punch to the side and then shoot your left straight to his eyes, gouging with all your fingers. Don't hesitate after your block, but make the motion one swift, seamless move from block to gouge.

3 sets, 10 reps — both sides

Clinch and Gouge

Use your heavy bag or a manikin-type bag for this one. Grab the bag as if you were clinching an attacker, jostling for a position of advantage. Pretend that he releases just enough pressure from your right arm for you to strike his eyes with your fingers. Your strike is successful because you don't need power for it to work. You just flick your phalanges into his eyeballs and watch him writhe in agony.

3 sets, 10 reps — both arms

Get Behind Him and Claw

Get behind your assailant whenever you can. Since there are countless ways to get behind an attacker, use your favorite for this exercise or consider the following easy method. Face your imaginary attacker. Pantomime pushing his right shoulder with your left hand and pulling his left shoulder with your right. Twist him around so that you are behind him, kick the back of his knee to lower him, and then reach over his head and rake your fingers across his eyes. Step back as you pull him down onto his back and finish him off with whatever techniques best apply.

2 sets, 10 reps — both sides

Sweep and Double Rake

Stand in a natural stance facing an imaginary attacker who is moving in with both his arms extended to push you. Move both of your arms in an arc, striking the outside of his right arm, pushing it and his left arm across his body. Now, reverse the arc motion with both hands, raking the assailant's eyes with your left, followed by your right. Make the clawing portion of the arc a fast whipping motion, a blur of 10 fingers ruining the attacker's day.

3 sets, 10 reps — both sides

Target Practice

To improve your accuracy, you need to create targets that represent an assailant's eyes. Striking the eyes requires more accuracy than punching the broad surface of an attacker's upper body. Use your imagination to make two little targets that are the height of an average man and as far apart as an average set of eyes. Here are some ideas.

Buttons   Glue two clothing buttons on a wall. You might even glue two or three sets, one at 5 feet six inches from the floor, another set at 6 feet and another at 6 feet 4 inches. Stand before the buttons and practice various ways to strike them.

3 sets, 15 reps – both sides

Metal rings   Go to a hardware store and buy two metal rings about the size of a quarter, or remove them from an old, three-ring school binder. Tape two of them together so that they are two or three inches apart, the same width as a set of eyes, and suspend them head high from the ceiling. Stand before them and practice single-finger strikes, multiple-finger strikes and thumb gouges.

3 sets, 15 reps – both sides

Eyeglass frames   Get an old pair of glasses and remove the lenses. Suspend them from the ceiling with string so that they hang head high. Stand before them and practice single finger strikes, multiple finger strikes and thumb gouges.

3 sets, 15 reps – both sides

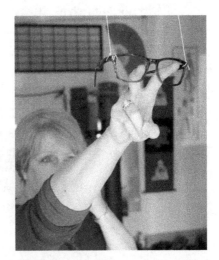

Paint-on eyes   Use White-out or some other type of marker and draw eyes on your heavy bag. Attack first with hand and foot blows, and then follow with finger strikes to the painted eyes. Or, attack the eyes first and follow up with punches and kicks.

3 sets, 10 reps – both sides

"The Cat"

Here is a goal for you. The late Master Gogen "The Cat" Yamaguchi, head of the Goju school of karate, was known for his extraordinary speed. One of his tricks was to hang a piece of cardboard by two slender threads and, standing before it, withdraw his hand into the sleeve of his gi. He would then shoot his hand out and withdraw it into his sleeve so lightening quick that observers were barely able to see the flicking movement. To the total amazement of those watching, the cardboard, which had not moved, suddenly had three holes in it.

FALLING

Many years ago, I read about a judo man who accidentally fell out of a second-story window (obviously, he was a clumsy judo man) but had the presence of mind to slap out as he landed on the sidewalk below (I would have been to busy screaming). Other than shattering the bones in his slapping arm, he was unhurt.

It's important to have at least a basic idea of how to fall. Some street fighters argue that in the street you are not going to be thrown to the sidewalk with a nice, clean judo throw that allows time and opportunity to slap out. They say that the assailant will probably crash to the sidewalk with you as he restrains your arms, keeping you from doing your break fall.

Important

Well, anything is possible in the street and their view is certainly valid. But also valid is that you just might have the opportunity to slap out, so wouldn't it be nice to know how? Another consideration, and an important one, is that knowing how to fall reduces your fear of it. People have a natural fear of losing their balance and crashing to the earth. So, the more you practice doing it, the more in control you will be of the situation, even when an attacker takes you to the ground against your will.

There are many falls in the arts of aikido, jujitsu and judo. If you have time and opportunity, learn them all. If you have neither, learn at least one method for falling on your face, one for falling on your back and one for falling on either side. Here are a few basic points to keep in mind until you get some expert instruction:

- Stay relaxed as you fall.
- Don't resist as you fall because that often causes you to land harder or more awkwardly.
- When falling backwards and to your side, tuck your chin to prevent hitting the ground with the back of your head.
- When falling forwards, lift your head a little and turn it to the side to prevent punching a hole in the ground with your nose.

Caution

- Never reach for the ground as you fall; it's a sure way to break a wrist or shoulder.
- Breathe out as you land to help reduce shock and maintain your normal breathing pattern

10 minutes, twice a week – include front, back and side falls

ANALYZE YOUR CLOTHING

This might seem like one of those training tips you see in books and magazines that no one ever practices, but I strongly urge you to experiment with these suggestions. Here is why it's important.

I joined the army three years after I began training in karate. I went from a loose-fitting karate uniform to loose-fitting fatigues. When I got to Vietnam and began getting into fights as a military policeman, the pants and shirt were not a problem, but those boots necessitated an adjustment. There is a big difference between kicking barefoot and kicking while wearing heavy, stiff, steel-toed jungle boots. Since I'm a slow learner, it took a few sprained ankles before I figured out that I needed to make an adjustment.

Two years later, I joined the police department. This time the uniform was considerably tighter than the karate and army uniforms and there was added weight, about 20 pounds of gear. Again, adjustments had to be made, and again, because of my slow learning problem, I got a couple of ripped-out inseams while being educated.

You probably practice and compete in one type of clothing, but on the street, where that buffed, drunk, fresh-out-of-prison con wants to clean your clock, you have on snug pants and a bulky coat. What about tonight when a bump from the back part of the house sends you scrambling out of bed and tiptoeing through the rooms in search of what made the sound? Will you be wearing boxers? A nightie? Nothing at all? Maybe you slip on a robe before you go out on your hunt. Have you ever practiced your techniques in your bathrobe and in those fuzzy pink slippers? What will you be wearing at work tomorrow? Have you tried your techniques while wearing that business suit or mini skirt? How about those sandals you wear to the beach? How about … You get the point.

Can you make a quick adjustment from how you do your techniques in your training uniform to how you need to do them in your regular clothing in the heat of a real battle? No, you cannot. Fighters who are convinced that they can are fooling themselves. It's similar to a friend of mine who refuses to wear a seat belt. "If I see that I'm going to get into an accident," she says, "I'll just quickly put it on." It doesn't work that way. You need to prepare in advance for a hot situation. Since you will be wearing clothing other than your training uniform, you must familiarize yourself as to how your techniques work, or don't work, while wearing them. Solo training is the perfect time to do it.

Train alone at least once a month wearing clothing other than your usual workout attire. Practice your bread and butter techniques, the ones you are most likely to use in a real fight, and create self-defense situations to see what you can and cannot do while wearing these clothes. Include these outfits.

Training Tip

- Street clothes
- Bathrobe
- Sandals
- Work clothes
- Boots
- Underwear (rethink training in the park)

KATA APPLICATIONS

There are far too many karate students who practice their kata without a clue as to the meaning. They perform them as if the arm and leg movements were part of a cheerleading routine or some new form of modern dance. They exhibit no fighting spirit, no concentration and no sense of intensity to their offensive and defensive movements. Sadly, it's not just colored belts who train and compete this way, but some black belts do, too. What has happened, especially with the black belts, is that they have allowed themselves to mentally get away from what they are supposed to be doing—fighting several attackers.

In *Fighter's Fact Book*, I discuss ways to bring a sense of fighting spirit and realism to your kata. Here is another way to do it that also helps to ingrain the real purpose of the movements in your mind. A nice side benefit is that you might even develop a few new techniques to add to your fighting repertoire.

Dissecting your Kata

Let's say the first combination move in your kata is a kick, block and counter punch. Pull out those three techniques so that you can analyze and practice them in front of a mirror. Let's say that the stance for those techniques is a deep and stylized one. First do two sets of 10 reps using the required stance to polish that part of your kata. Then adjust the stance—bringing your feet closer together and standing a little higher—to make it more functional for sparring and self-defense. Now, do 2 sets of 10 reps of the kick, block and counter punch from that stance. Go through your entire kata pulling out sections, particularly blocks and counters. Practice them just as they are performed in the kata and then make them workable for reality fighting. If there are some that are workable just as they are, you won't need to make an adjustment.

Those fancy smancy moves   But what can you do with those flamboyant, over-the-top techniques seen in modern kata, such as back flips, somersaults and aerial cartwheels? Obviously (it should be obvious, anyway), these things are not functional in tournaments or street fighting, though unfortunately they are needed to win in today's tough kata competition.

For this translation exercise, you have two choices: You can ignore the showmanship techniques and skip over to the next functional ones, or you can see if there are any parts in the fancy stuff that you can use. For example, if after you land from that aerial cartwheel you execute a punch, kick combination, pull out the punch and kick and work just on them. With that handspring, see if you can pick out the techniques that lead up to the spring or those techniques that immediately follow.

The value of kata has become a controversial subject in recent years. If your style does them but you don't like doing them, make the best of your training using this analytical exercise.

DOUBLE-END BAG

The double-end bag, sometimes called the "goofy bag," is mentioned in other places in this book as a supplemental exercise to other drills. Let's take a look now at how you can spend a few minutes whacking it to improve your footwork, body movement and commitment to hitting a moving target.

Training Tip

It's important to secure your bag to remove excessive play; it confuses your timing when the bag flies 15 feet away each time it's struck. Tighten it down (try attaching a rope to the top portion and an elastic cord on the bottom) to reduce its swing to 12 to 18 inches. Adjust the rope and elastic so the bag is about level with your head, give or take a couple inches.

Work the Outside

The double-end bag is great for working the so-called outside area, a place from where you hit with fully extended jabs, reverse punches, backfists, hooks, checks, slaps, palm-heel strikes, forearms, finger gouges, rakes, and ridgehand strikes. Use your footwork to move forward, shuffle away, sidestep, diagonal step and scoot forwards and backwards. Use your checks and sweep-type blocks to stop the returning bag from hitting you as you move to better connect with another blow. For example, execute a backfist and then as the bag returns, hit it with a reverse punch. As it returns again, step diagonally and claw it as it passes. Step into its return path and throw a quick jab and reverse punch. If at any time you get caught off guard and bopped in the nose, that is a good thing. Learn from it. What did you do wrong? Correct it and move on.

Get Close

Move in closer this time and hit it with an elbow strike. When it comes back, headbutt it away and elbow it again when it returns. Although the bag is too high to knee strike, knee the air below the bag and follow with an elbow strike to the bag. You are close, so you need to be alert and fast since the bag returns quickly.

Move In or Move Out

In this last phase, begin at the outside range as you did in the first phase, throwing jabs, reverses and so on, but then use your footwork to close in and finish with elbows to the bag, knees to the air and headbutts to the bag. You can also start at close range with elbows and headbutts, and then move outside as you punch and strike. Look for opportunities to throw kicks, too. Kick at the air under the bag and follow with hand techniques on the bag.

How Hard to Hit

Many fighters don't hit the double-end bag with full-power blows because they are working only on their accuracy, timing and *Workout Tip* footwork. If your bag can tolerate full power, go ahead and clobber away, but not until you feel comfortable with all the other attributes you are training for. If you have a lightweight double-end bag and feel that a series of hard blows might snap the cord and send it out the window, do your hard blows on the heavy bag instead. One way to train is to use lighter blows on the double-end bag for 10 minutes and then hard blows on the heavy bag for 10.

The double-end bag can be a real challenge at first, but don't give up. Your coordination will show itself within two or three workouts.

Double-end bag: 20-30 minutes, nonstop

Combination bags: 30 minutes — double-end bag: 10 min; heavy bag: 5 min; double-end bag, 5 min; heavy bag, 10 min

KNEE-LIFT JAM

This is a popular tournament technique that has been around for a long time. I used it on several occasions as a police officer when I had to charge at a suspect who was threatening with kicks or some type of club. My purpose was to jam the threat while reducing my body targets. Once I was on him, I used my hands to jam his closest arm, spin him around and take him to the ground. There are solid advantages to the move and a couple of risks, but when executed with explosiveness, your rate of success will be high.

In sparring, the knee-lift jam is great for closing on an opponent who is preparing to attack, such as when he lifts his leg to kick or cocks back his backfist. Since his thoughts are on what he is going to do to you, he is more vulnerable to your sudden offensive jam. For example, when he lifts his leg to kick, jam his leg with your knee or shin, check his closest arm and drive a punch into whatever target is hanging out there.

The knee-lift jam can be incorporated into most gap-closing stepping methods, though probably the ones used most often are the skip, shuffle step and crossover step. With all of them, it's important to lean your upper body 5-10 degrees toward the opponent as you charge. This ensures that your momentum is moving forward and your balance is stable when you clash with your opponent's force. Here is how to knee jam using three of the basic steps that have been discussed previously.

Skip Step

There are two methods of skipping forward from your fighting stance. The first is to lift your front knee and skip forward on your rear foot. You travel only a few inches but you move quickly. The second way is to raise your rear knee, move it past your front leg and then skip forward on your lead foot to close the distance. It's a tad slower, but you can cover a couple of feet with a lot of momentum.

Rear knee jam: 2 sets, 15 reps – both sides
Front knee jam: 2 sets, 15 reps – both sides

Replacement Step

From your fighting stance, close the distance by stepping forward with your rear foot to the heel of your lead foot, and then lifting your lead knee to jam.

2 sets, 15 reps

Crossover Step

From your fighting stance, lift your rear knee and bring it forward past your front leg and jam your invisible opponent with it. This is similar to the skip step using the rear leg. The difference is that you don't skip forward with this variation.

2 sets, 15 reps – both sides

As the assailant, Professor Tim Delgman, prepares to kick, I execute a crossover step and jam his kicking leg with what was my rear leg.
I then follow through by jamming his lead arm and punching him in the middle.

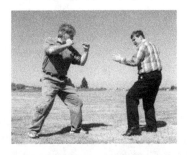

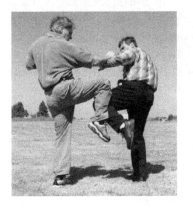

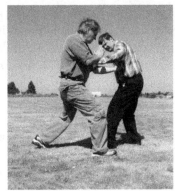

SOLO TRAINING WITH A PARTNER

Partners

Can you really train alone and with another person at the same time? Yes, sort of. Let's say you and your training partner want to train together, but you also want to spend some training time on one or more things specific to your needs. If your partner also wants to work on a couple of things by himself during your session, you have yourself the perfect date, as long as the two of can agree as to how you are going to do it. One way is for you and your partner to train together for the first half of your session and then you both train alone the second half. Or, you can start out training alone and then finish the session training together. For example, you can spar for 20 minutes, then for the next 30 minutes, the two of you practice solo to solidify those sparring techniques that worked especially well, and to work on those that didn't. To round out the hour, the two of you spar again for another 10 minutes.

Maybe you both have a belt examine coming up, a test that includes kata as well as punching and kicking drills with a partner. Spend half of your training session working together polishing the drills and then finish your session by separating to opposite sides of the room to work on your individual katas.

Alone, you can train in just about any small space, but you need a larger space for two of you. One possibility is to get access to your school when there are no classes in session. My old training buddy and I did that and found it perfect because after we worked together, I had ample room to do my forms and he had access to the heavy bags to work on his power. But if you can't get into your school, consider your backyard, a neighborhood grade school, a garage, an old building.

If you have trouble getting yourself motivated to train alone, doing it with a partner is a good way to progressively introduce yourself to the idea.

COPING WITH INJURIES

If you have been training in the martial arts for more than a week, you know that injuries are part of the experience, though most of the time, they are not so significant that they keep you from training. A jammed finger can be taped to a healthy one, a crumpled toe can be covered with a shoe, and so on. But ever so often you get one that sidelines you for a couple weeks, a couple months or longer. It's sort of a cruel joke perpetrated by fate that the more serious injuries always occur at a time when you are making your best progress.

This old horse has received just about every injury imaginable. I've had lots and lots of broken fingers, toes, sprained wrists, tweaked elbows and twisted ankles. My most serious injuries were a broken knee, damaged larynx, broken rib and a crushed kidney. What I learned from all of these unpleasantries is that it's still possible to do some kind of training. For example, when my knee was in a foot-to-groin cast for several months, I practiced my punches and backfists while sitting in a chair. I lifted weights while sitting and lying on a bench, and I worked arm and upper body stretching while propped on crutches. When a side kick broke my rib, pain and doctor's orders prohibited me from doing all upper body movement for the first few weeks. So I did zillions of horse-stance squats, one-legged squats, stair climbing, power walks, calf raises and some carefully controlled weight exercises for my arms.

When you get injured, establish a mindset that you are not going to sit around and feel sorry for yourself, eat garbage food and wait for nature to heal you. Instead, immediately begin thinking about how you are going to come out of the injury stronger. For example, if you jammed your toes, plan to spend your time drilling on hand techniques. If you blew a thumb joint, apply your energy to improving your kicks. Consider developing skill with a weapon. One of the benefits of my months recuperating from my trashed knee is that I became quite good at fighting with a cane.

Bite the Bullet

Okay, you got injured. It hurts. It looks to be a long-term injury and you can see all your hard training going down the drain. You are sooo depressed. Well, snap out of it! You grieved for a couple days (athletes are big on self pity), now it's time to get positive. There is always something you can do while you heal, even if it's just squeezing a hand gripper. Figure out what it is that you can do to improve another phase of your training without aggravating your injury, and get to it.

And please. Stop whining.

A SHORT, EFFECTIVE SET OF ABDOMINAL EXERCISES

Hard stomach muscles are not just for looking good at the beach (although if we are truthful with ourselves, looking good at the beach is pretty darn important). As a martial artist, strong abs support your lower back, add stability to your balance and add power to all your techniques. You owe it to yourself to have a strong midsection, and you owe it to the art you represent not to have a gut hanging over your belt. You don't have to have a visible six pack of ab muscles, but you do have to have power there. Here is one excellent way to get it.

There is a small controversy in bodybuilding circles as to whether it's a good idea to use weight resistance with abdominal exercises. The con side claims that resistance exercise builds a thick, muscular waist, which is not a good thing for those interested in the visual sport of bodybuilding. The pros argue that weight resistance does not build large abdominal muscles, but rather hardens and shapes them.

Workout
Tip

Several years ago I competed in a bodybuilding contest. I trained like a mad man at the gym each night until I barely had enough energy to drive home. Since burning out hundreds of crunches and leg lifts was draining my energy reserve and affecting the poundage I needed to lift to add size to my other muscles, I decided to experiment with crunches with a barbell plate on my chest. I read somewhere that the abdominal muscles respond the same way as other muscles respond to exercise. You don't do 300 repetitions of barbell curls, so why do 300 reps of crunches? That made sense to me, so I grabbed a 10-pound plate, held it to my chest and did four sets of 15 reps of crunches.

I was intensely sore the next day, something I hadn't felt in a long time, though I was regularly doing 200 to 300 crunches on abdominal days. Within a couple weeks, I found that the 10-pound plate was too light, so I added another 10 pounds. A week after that, I was doing crunches with a 25-pound plate. Two months later, a 50-pound plate. I decided not to add any more weight because I didn't think it was necessary, and it was getting hard to balance the weight on my chest.

I entered the physique contest with the best six pack of abs I've ever had. I almost felt as if I were cheating since I didn't rep out hundreds of crunches and leg raises like the other competitors. All I did were 3 or 4 sets of 10 to 15 reps.

Here are three exercises that work the upper and lower abs and those between the front and sides.

Upper Abs

Lie on the floor, feet tucked up next to your rear. Place a barbell plate of your choice on your chest and cross your arms over it to keep it in place. Point your chin up, flex your ab muscles and lift your head and upper back until your shoulder blades are four to six inches off the floor. Return to the floor and do another rep.
2 sets, 10 reps

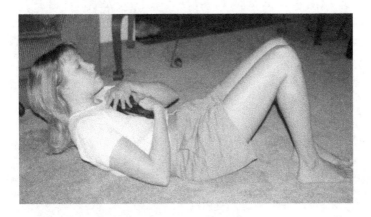

Upper and Lower Abs

Lie on your back and hold a 2-5-pound dumbbell between your feet and a barbell plate on your chest. Slowly draw both knees toward your chest while curling your head and shoulders off the floor. Point your chin high throughout the movement and forcibly flex your abs. Breathe out as you come up, hold at the top for one second and then slowly lower yourself back to the floor. For added tension, do not allow the weight between your feet to touch the floor until the last rep is completed. This places added tension on those hard-to-work lower abs.

2 sets, 10 reps

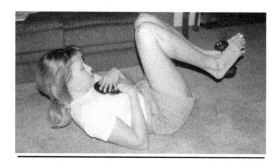

Begin with your head on the floor, your legs extended with a barbell plate on your chest and a dumbbell held between your feet. Lift your head and shoulders as you simultaneously draw your knees toward your chest as pictured. Do 2 sets, 10 reps

Upper Abs and Oblique Abs

Lie on your back with your knees bent so that your feet are about half way to your rear. With both hands, grasp your favorite barbell plate, 5 to 10 pounds at first, and extend your arms so the plate is just above your groin (be careful). Keeping your arms extended, lift your head and shoulders off the floor as you slowly twist your torso to the left. The plate will end up near the outside of your left knee. Lower yourself and repeat, this time twisting to your right, so that the weight ends up outside your right knee. Continue alternating the reps.

2 sets, 10 reps

When you first sit up in bed the morning after the first time through this ab routine, you will have unkind thoughts about me. And you may hear your stomach muscles scream.

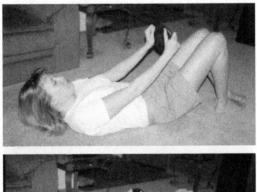

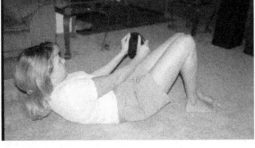

Begin on your back with your legs bent as you hold a barbell plate over your groin area . Lift your head and shoulders and extend your arms so that the barbell plate is near the outside of your left knee. Lower your head back to the floor as you move the plate back over your groin. Without stopping, repeat on the other side.

7

MENTAL TRAINING

Before we examine such important mental attributes as developing a training and fighting philosophy, ways to use mental imagery to improve your self-defense skills and how to replace old negative internal tapes with positive ones, let's take a quick look at how your training helps your mind stay sharp as a tack.

EXERCISE IS GOOD FOR YOUR BRAIN

There is no argument that working out is good for your body: it makes you feel good and look good (Californians, say that looking good is more important than feeling good). But working out regularly is also good for the ol' grey matter. It improves your mood, self-esteem and even your ability to think clearly. Scientists are continually researching new ways that exercise improves your mental and emotional state.

Exercise produces endorphins.

These are nature's natural drugs that are released when you train hard. They make you feel good, almost "high," and block pain.

It makes you feel good about yourself.

A good solo workout leaves you feeling elated that you have accomplished something that is good for you.

It raises your testosterone level.

A hard training session, especially if you have incorporated weight training, will improve your mood as a result of an elevated testosterone level.

It releases antidepressant chemicals.

Your hard workout releases goodies like dopamine and serotonin, which elevates your mood.

Reduces anger and tension.

A good solo session can relieve all the anger and tension that builds throughout the day.

Training aerobically helps your thinking.

Those 20 - 60 minute aerobic workouts may leave you sweaty and winded, but they also improve circulation to your brain.

It might make you smarter.

Your workouts will not only reduce the loss of brain function as you age, but new studies show that it may actually help you develop new brain cells.

It is a form of moving meditation.

A good solo workout will take your brain away from brooding on that bad grade you got in school or the lousy day you had at work.

It improves your sleep.

Consistent training may improve the quality and length of your sleep.

Okay, now that you see how physical exercise can get your grey matter in the pink, let's look at a few ways you can use that gray stuff to help improve your fighting ability.

YOUR BEST WEAPON

In the process of developing your punches, kicks, and jumps, it's important that you don't neglect your greatest weapon -- your mind. Of course you use it to think about target and technique selection, timing, and how to best use your body to deliver your blows with speed, power and accuracy. But there is more to incorporating your mind in your fighting art than just using it to execute proper physical technique.

Develop a Personal Philosophy

It's important to develop a personal philosophy about your training and self-defense so that you have a clear direction when temptation, fatigue and fear are clouding and distorting your view of reality. If you don't have a personal philosophy, you are like a rudderless ship bouncing around on the waves. Your direction is unclear. Your training goals are fuzzy and your thoughts of when to fight and when not to fight are vague. Use your time alone to develop a plan of action so that you know where you are going and what you are going to do when you get there.

i
Important

Use your solo time   Keep in mind that your training alone time does not always have to be physical. This is good news for those times you want to do something, but the thought of throwing one more kick or punch sends you to the kitchen to cut off a big piece of cake and then to the living room to find the television remote. Know your body well enough so you can tell the difference between when you are being lazy and when your body is telling you to give it a rest.

When your body is truly crying for relief, reward it with some down time, but instead of watching television, spend the time thinking about your fighting art and how your personal philosophy relates to it. You can do this in your easy chair, while lying in a hammock under a tree, driving in your car, waiting for the bus, walking in your neighborhood or when simply staring out the window at the pattering rain.

Advantages to this kind of training are that you don't get sweaty or winded and no one is kicking you in the face. But the biggest advantage is that you begin to develop a mental edge that guides you in training, competing, or a self-defense encounter.

Your Training Philosophy

I have been calling it "your personal" philosophy because it's just that: Your way of thinking. I'm not going to be presumptuous here and tell you what to think. Instead, bear with me while I give you my philosophy. If you like it, you can use it. Or, you can add to it, or delete some or all of it and create your own. What is important is that your philosophy works for you.

There are three parts to my personal philosophy of training and they are all simple:

- I do lots of reps.
- I don't prearrange my responses.
- I always keep in mind that when I'm not training, my opponent is.

Allow me to elaborate.

Reps   In *Fighter's Fact Book*, I browbeat the reader as to the importance of doing reps, physically pounding them out and mentally visualizing them. It's important that you accept the fact that you need to do thousands and thousands of reps to truly master a technique. This doesn't mean you have to sit in horse stance and punch mindlessly for hours. I trained that way in a traditional system for several years, and while I developed a good punch, I discovered later that there are many other drills and exercises in which I can do reps, but do so while developing practical applications and while keeping my sanity. Use your learning to develop all kinds of ways to do reps.

How many: Here is what Instructor Marc MacYoung says about the value of practicing reps. "In the Orient, they tell you to do a technique 10,000 times. After 100 reps you're totally confused. At 500 reps you are still concentrating on getting better, and at one thousand you impress yourself with how good you are. At two thousand reps you are blazing through it, and at three thousand you are convinced you are so good you could have beat Bruce Lee. Around four thousand reps you are getting bored, and at five thousand you are thoroughly bored. Around six thousand you are so bored that you begin to look at what you are doing just for something to do. At seven thousand reps you start thinking that there are more things you can do with the technique than what you originally thought. Around eight thousand, you are so wrapped up in all the possibilities that you don't even remember that you are bored. At 10,000 reps, you finally understand all the implications of the technique."

Training Tip

We are the Mc Donald's generation, meaning, we want it now. But that does not work with the martial arts, which is all about training and doing kazillions of reps. Ingrain that in your mind, and you will inch ever closer to mastery.

Prearranged responses One time, I was talking with a high-ranking karate teacher about technique. I asked how he taught his students to respond to an arms-pinned bear hug from the front. He looked puzzled for a log moment and then scratched his head. "Uh, let's see. That one's on page 18 in our technique binder. Um . . ."

Well, let's just hope my friend has time to thumb through his technique binder when he gets attacked in an alley.

I never teach specific, set responses to a given attack because there are too many possible variables. For example, say you memorize a response to an attacker's front choke as the two of you stand in the middle of the room. You practice and practice until you have your response down as smooth as a whistle. But what if in a real situation the attacker pushes you against a wall as he chokes you, or he bends you over a railing as he squeezes the air out of your throat? It's quite possible, since you have practiced only one variation, that you will not do anything other than gasp for air.

It's far more effective to have one or two responses to a given attack and then analyze them as to how they are applied, with some modification, in a variety of situations. Let's consider the basic tackle, where an attacker charges you with the intent to wrap his arms around your waist, hips or legs. Many fighters err by training to defend only against that point where the attackers' arms are wrapped around their legs. It's okay to practice that, but it's not the only stage in the attack that should be studied. What if you have the opportunity to defend against it at another stage in the attack? For example . . .

Training Tip

• From five feet away when the attacker starts to crouch and raise his arms

• From three feet away when he is crouched low and his arms are reaching

• When his hands are just a few inches away from you

• As he shoots in toward your legs

• As his hands touch you

• As his arms encircle you.

• As he lifts you up

• As you land on your back

Since there are many stages to the tackle, your training is incomplete if you practice just one, preset response. But let's say you are on the ball and you have practiced responding to the tackle in all the stages listed. That is good, but don't settle back all comfy and say, "Okay, this is the technique I will use in this stage and this is what I will do in that stage." That is a no-no because there are so many variables.

For example, the attacker might try to tackle you on stairs, on wet grass or in a cluttered room (once, a monster of a guy tried to tackle me on a bridge that spans the churning, angry waters of the Willamette River). The attacker might out weigh you by 50 pounds or he might be a wiry and quick little guy.

To reiterate the point: Don't get comfortable and settle on one, absolute response.

Here is what Instructor Kenneth Smith says, "Situation dictates application. An attacker will not move or stand exactly the way you want or the way you have practiced in the dojo. The position of your body to his, where your weight is in relation to his line of attack, and even your mood at that particular moment, will all dictate how you respond and where you will strike back. Do not even try to plan a defense in advance. Just wait for the proper moment and respond naturally and instinctively, like an echo to a sound."

Kenneth talked about the dangers of too many responses: "It is impossible to respond naturally and instinctively when your mind is occupied with hundreds of separate, preprogrammed responses. Instead of overwhelming yourself with a voluminous catalog of techniques, simply pick two or three of your favorite responses and practice them to as near perfection as you can, then learn to adapt them to any and all types of attacks."

My approach is to practice a response repetitiously - and then forget it. Using the tackle attack as an example, I have my students perform several reps of one or two responses when the attacker is in the first stage of the attack. Then we move to the next stage and do one or two responses over and over for it, always pushing for speed and power. We continue in this fashion all the way through the various stages.

While it's important to practice at least two responses to a situation, be careful not to engrave them in stone. Don't say to yourself, "This is what I would do if a guy tackled me." Instead, contemplate a tackle's complexity and then practice in all stages of it, including ways to adapt your two or three responses to variables.

I encourage you to spend your solo time thinking in this fashion about all kinds of attacks, and always keep in mind that even a seemingly simple attack, such as a roundhouse punch to your nose, can have many variables.

Keep training   My other philosophy is to do something toward my fighting art at least five days a week. Some days I train hard physically, other days I research a new training idea or technique in my library of books, videos and magazines. This is a philosophy I started years ago as a police officer. I always held the thought that on those days I skipped karate training or lifting weights, there was a big, nasty tattooed guy in prison lifting hard and practicing getting out of my police holds.

Important

If you are a competitor and you want to skip a day of training to go hang out with the guys, think about your opponent hammering the heavy bag, a bag with your picture on it. And when you skip your kata practice, think about your opponent fine tuning his kata and imagining his trophy, the one you are not going to win.

If your slant is self-defense and you sluff off on your training, know that at the same time there is a street punk out there thinking about his next caper, the one where he beats his victim just for the fun of it before he takes his money. Or think about those tough guys you always see shooting pool in bars and loitering on street corners, the guys with buffed muscles and fighting knowledge garnered from the streets. You innocently bump into one and he is in your face accusing you of wanting to start something. Think about them on those days you skip your training.

To sum up. My training philosophy is simple:

1. I do lots of reps in a variety of ways to not only work my muscles, but to imprint the action in my brain so that the physical and mental form a powerful link.

2. I never plan an exact response since I don't know exactly how I'm going to be attacked.

3. I seldom miss training, even if it's only to read a martial arts magazine or ponder my personal philosophy.

Now, spend time thinking about your philosophy as it relates to training.

Fighting Philosophy

You can listen to what your instructor teaches you about his philosophy of fighting and you can listen to what other students believe, but in the end you must formulate a philosophy that works for you. For example, consider these questions. What does it take to make you react physically to a threatening situation? Would there ever be a time you would not fight, no matter how extreme the circumstances? Have you thought what it would be like to beat someone to death? Actually kill someone with your karate techniques?

Here are a couple of concepts for you to ponder during your solo time, concepts that I have thought out and developed a philosophy for. If you have not taken the time to think out your personal fighting philosophy, use mine as a foundation to get you started. Let's begin with examining the killer instinct and then consider how to develop a philosophy for fighting intimidating looking people.

Killer Instinct   For the moment, forget about sport karate. Forget about the trend of using karate movements for aerobic conditioning, or your goal of passing your next belt exam. These are all important, but set them aside so you can think about only one thing—fighting for your life. Take a moment to mentally create a scenario that is so grave that you are legally justified to take the attacker's life. Really ponder that thought. Don't just say empty words to yourself or get caught up in bravado, but really think about the hard, cold reality of killing another human. Do you have what it takes to do it? Could you beat an assailant to death with your hands and feet? You know, using your body weapons to kill someone is not as "clean" as shooting a person from several feet away. With a gun you cannot "feel" the person you are killing. But you sure can with your hands and feet.

Here are a couple of questions that are often pondered and debated. Are the streets of American cities, large cities in particular, war zones as some people contend? Most street people who hang out on the streets, such as homeless people fighting to survive every day, so-called innocent people who are victimized by muggers, rapists, thieves, and the violently mentally ill, and police officers who

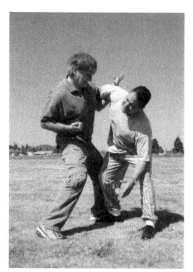

Have you considered whether you could take a life if you had no other choice? After trapping the assailant's arm, I drive a powerful uppercut into his throat.

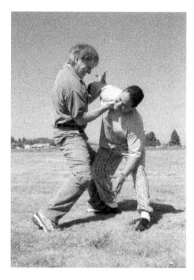

struggle daily to keep the peace, agree that there is a war in progress. Other people, who have not had the same experiences as these people, are more likely to argue that the streets of our American cities are just fine. Some of them even believe that criminals, those who physically attack the unwary, are poor unfortunates acting out because they were abused as children or because they didn't have the same opportunities growing up as others did. There are lots of opinions on the subject because people argue from a place that has been formed by their experiences.

While it may be interesting to argue, debate and study these issues, if an assailant is trying to hurt me or a loved one, my primary concern is to survive the moment, not think about the psychological or sociological reason he is doing it. My only thought and objective when engaged in a life and death struggle with an attacker are to give my all to the fight. I must fight to win. I must fight to stop the assailant, even if it means killing him.

I believe that everyone has a killer instinct, even a guy who wears bow ties, carries pocket protectors and uses tape to hold his glasses together. Such a guy may look meek and mild, but when the right situation arises – such as when someone slaps his mother or pulls food from his kid's hands -- he will fight and do so with awesome ferociously.

If you are a martial artist who trains for street self-defense, it's important that you understand that the killer instinct resides within you, and that it will make you stronger, faster and resistant to pain. Knowing that it's there, will make it easier to draw it out of your mind, and do so in an instant.

Here is a method that I have taught for many years that helps some people bring their killer instinct to the surface. Admittedly, it's controversial, and one that not everyone is comfortable with. If it's not for you, I encourage you to seek other ways.

Dehumanize your assailant: Mentally dehumanizing the enemy is a device that has been used by soldiers throughout history in order for them to fight with intensity and to kill. I'm not suggesting that you look at your assailant through eyes filled with racial hatred, or with ethnic, religious, sexual orientation, or gender prejudice. On the other hand, I'm not saying that you shouldn't take that approach. When you are in a fight for your life, you cannot do so with limitations, you cannot hold back because of morals, a sense of humanity, religious reasons, fear of arrest or of being sued.

Arguably, the greatest reason to hold back is because of religious reasons, and if that is your reason, you need to be aware that any psychological glitch that interferes with your life and death struggle, dramatically increases your chance of losing. Don't misunderstand and think that I'm telling not to be religious. I'm not. I'm saying that if this is your belief, you need to think about it as it relates to your personal philosophy of self-defense, especially a situation in which you or the person you are protecting may be killed if you do not act.

I don't want to take a life, but if the situation is so grave that I am absolutely convinced that I will I die if I lose, my philosophy is that I owe it myself and to my family to use whatever personal psychological ploy that is available to help me survive the moment. If that means I must see the assailant as a rabid, junkyard dog, or some other nonpolitically correct image, so be it. If that philosophy is offensive to others, too bad. It has gotten me through some pretty nasty alleyways, and it's why I am able to sit here today and pound the keyboard.

Granted, this is not a topic I would discuss with my grandmother or with nice folks at a church social. These people would probably not understand because fighting to the death is far removed from their reality. But as a martial artist, a warrior, it is my reality. My philosophy is this: If I am attacked with deadly viciousness or an innocent person in my presence is attacked with deadly viciousness, I will respond with the same. I do not want to kill, but if I have no option . . .

I sincerely hope that you never have to call upon your killer instinct. However, it's critical that you contemplate its possibility. Spend solo time thinking about it and developing a philosophy that works for you.

When you are in a fight for your life, you cannot do so with limitations.

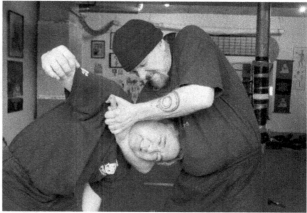

FIGHTING THE BIG GUYS

As a police officer for 29 years, I fought many people, some consideraly bigger than I, some smaller. Although the big ones were sometimes visually intimidating - especially those with bulging veins on their forehead and tattoos of pittbulls on their necks - they were no tougher than the smaller people. Yes, they were often stronger than I, and their mass made them a challenge, but as far as fighting skill, none of them stand out in my mind from any of the average-sized suspects. In fact, when I reflect on the major brawls I've had, the ones that immediately pop into mind are those I had with average-sized people or below average.

Mentally Prepare for the Big Guys

If you have not prepared yourself mentally, a big bruiser of a guy can easily psyche you out. Imagine one of those 280-pound professional wrestlers screaming in your face. Whenever I'm asked what I would do against a giant of human flesh and muscle like a World Wrestling Federation wrestler/entertainer, I say, "I'd jam my index finger up to my third knuckle in his eyeball, and then I would run like a Cheetah on an African plain."

A policeman friend of mine got too close to a big, mean guy and the giant picked him up as if he were a child. The officer managed not to panic, and crammed his thumb in the big ape's eye socket and wiggled it around like he was stirring tea with a spoon. The big guy, who outweighed the diminutive officer by 150 pounds, dropped him like a hot potato and later complained of police brutality.

My point is this: A big guy may have Buick-sized arms and a neck larger than your chest, but he is still a human, and humans have vulnerable targets: eyes, throat, groin, fingers, shins, and toes.

This philosophy holds true in competition, too. I once attended a seminar taught by world champion point karate and full-contact fighter Joe Lewis. He advised us to never be intimidated by the color of an opponent's belt. He said that although you may be a pink belt and the mean looking guy in front of you has slashes all over his black one, he still has only two arms and two legs, and there is only so many things he can do with them.

Important

Instructor Ken Smith says this about facing a big guy. "Don't be intimidated by the size of your assailant. Look at him as if you were staring straight through him, and focus your mind on just one thing and one thing only -- escape! Narrow your eyes as you look through him, and ever so subtly flare your nostrils, which will deepen and slow your breathing. These two actions will help steady your thoughts and calm your nerves."

Smith continues: "Human beings seem to think that bigger and stronger will automatically mean more dangerous. But, some of the most deadly creatures in nature are the smallest and most delicate. The Black Mamba is a good example. It is a little snake whose bite can kill a man in just a few minutes. Just because an assailant appears intimidating, does not mean that he is any more or any less of a threat than a smaller man. After all, a punch is still a punch, no matter who throws it. If you deflect it, rather than try to block its trajectory with brute force, you will only need about ten ounces of strength to redirect it. The amount of power behind the punch is not important. It only takes 10 ounces to redirect ANY attack. So, don't be concerned with the size or apparent ferocity of your opponent. Merely observe the angle and direction of his attack, and deal with it appropriately."

I encourage you to spend time contemplating the issue of visually intimidating opponents so that you are less threatened by a competitor's size, belt color, clothing or body adornments. Develop a philosophy that allows you to see the person as only a problem to be dealt with, a problem that you can successfully handle. Tell yourself that his big fists and feet *can* be blocked. His neck tattoos and multi-striped black belt are only adornments. He is still a person, and the bigger he is, the louder the noise he'll make when he hits the ground.

Although specific ways to fight a really large person is beyond the scope of this section, I don't want to leave you hanging, and I'll resist being a smart aleck by saying, "You fight a very, very big person very, very carefully." Instead, I offer here a couple of ideas for you to consider. They are both taught by Joe Lewis and they work well.

Don't Let Him set Himself

Lewis teaches that the only time a person is dangerous, whether he is big or small, is when he sets himself, which is defined as that partial second just prior to the launch of his attack. To keep him from doing this, keep moving, using busy footwork, body motion, feints, and broken rhythm to keep him confused and unable to attack with those big, hairy fists of his.

Important

Hit His Limbs

I discuss and illustrate this second method of Lewis's, in *Fighter's Fact Book*. In short, rather than getting inside the big guy where he can do lots of bad things to you, stay on his outside and work on his limbs. Stay in motion so that he can't set himself to attack, and punch his forearms, upper arms and the back of hands. With your feet, attack his thighs, knees, shins and ankles. Once he is injured and weakened, that is when you slip inside and hit his throat, groin and eyes to weaken him even further. In competition, hit his arms (leg shots are illegal) to distract him as you work your way inside.

I've barely scratched the surface of Lewis's teachings and I encourage you to seek out his writings and attend his seminars where he elaborates on these concepts.

It's All in the Mind

Intimidation is a state of mind. An opponent, whether in the street, in competition or in class, is intimidating only if you allow him to be. When you allow an image or symbol—muscles, tattoos, belt color—to intimidate you, you create another opponent to deal with. But if you think of your opponent, one who happens to have these images and symbols, as an opponent with arms and legs who can do only so much with them, the intimidation factor is reduced or eliminated. Symbols cannot hurt you. Big muscles, or the presence of a weapon, need to be taken into account, just as you need to take into account an opponent's exceptional speed or trickiness. But taking them into account is not the same as being intimidated by them.

Don't wait until you are facing an intimidating guy to think about all this; instead, contemplate it in advance. Use your solo time to think about my philosophy as I've discussed it here, or use it as a base from which you build your own. Once you have found one that works for you, intimidating opponents will no longer seem intimidating and you will have crossed a big hurdle.

IMAGERY

I have discussed mental imagery in several of my books because it's a powerful training device that cannot be ignored. Performance in any endeavor is largely dependant upon mental preparation and psychological strength. Just as you prepared for competition by practicing your sparring and kata, you must also prepare yourself mentally.

Most often, mental imagery is practiced after you induce a state of deep relaxation. You find a quiet, comfortable place and begin with deep breathing and whatever mental device you have found that gets your mind and body calmed and deeply relaxed. This condition makes you more susceptible to the positive images that you create—such as a perfectly executed roundhouse kick or a flawless kick/punch combination—images that later will be duplicated in your physical performance.

THE WORLD IS YOUR DOJO

Although inducing relaxation prior to mental imagery practice is the best method to visualize, you can still practice in other settings—work place, school, bus, car, street corner, movie theater, restaurant—places where people and "training equipment" are already provided for your imagined self-defense scenarios.

A martial arts instructor I know teaches that we should not shut off our training the moment we step off the mat or leave the school. "The whole world is your dojo," he said. "Everywhere and everyone are involved in your training, even when you sleep." Whether you take it to that extreme is up to you. Personally, I'm not going to walk around in a constant state of training; life is too short and there are too many other interesting things to do. But on those occasions when I do want to get in a little solo training and I'm out in public, I have to agree with that instructor: The whole world is a dojo. Here are two examples.

My Friend the Assassin

I have a friend who makes the whole world his firing range. There is a risk in my relating this story because every reader is going to hear its meaning differently. Some will think that what he does is a great idea, while others will think he is one sick puppy. If you fall into the latter group, understand that this has helped him survive as a cop in a tough city and it has helped make him the master, nationally-ranked shooter that he is.

Although David is retired now from police work, he is still a competitive shooter. He has won so many trophies that if they were all melted down they could be remade into a fleet of oversized American cars. He still competes at least two weekends a month and practices nearly every day. Once he nearly cut off his trigger finger with an electric saw, but the next weekend he was at the range competing, shooting with his middle finger and winning a second-place trophy.

David rode a bus every day to work, a 15-minute trip during which he often practiced shooting fellow passengers. Although he had won hundreds of shooting awards, he had never fired his weapon at a live, blood-filled person. Paper targets, yes. People, no. So he took advantage of his bus trip to get in a little practice on some of the passengers.

My friend usually sat in the back of the bus where he would eyeball a guy sitting in one of those sideways seats near the driver. The guy's race or age didn't matter to David, nor did it matter whether he was a homeless person or a powerful executive on the way to one of the big office buildings downtown. If he was in David's imaginary sites, he was going to get shot.

With his hands folded serenely in his lap and using only his imagination, David superimposed the front sights of his favorite gun over the selected guy's ear or forehead. It was important to get the sites lined up perfectly and to hold the imaginary weapon motionless. Hold, breathe out gently, squeeze the trigger . . . Kaboom!

If someone even noticed my unassuming friend, all he saw was a guy who looked half asleep in his seat just like most of the other passengers. There was no way the observer could tell by looking at David that he had just shot a passenger sitting in the front of the bus and that he was now moving his imaginary gunsites over to another person.

As I said, some people might find this exercise sick, but David could care less. He knows that statistically, competition shooters do not do well in real shootings where their targets are breathing and shooting back. He believes that his solo training on his bus helps him prepare for shooting at a human target. David retired after 25 years as a street cop and though he drew his weapon on several occasions in the line of duty, he was never forced to fire it. For that he is grateful. He still competes today, adding trophy after trophy to his collection.

And he still rides the bus.

Imagine Punching, Kicking & Sweeping Innocent People

I have used David's training method for years and have found it highly beneficial. I do not use a gun on innocent people but I do use my martial arts. It's an easy way to practice and I can do it anywhere at any time, and no one has a clue what I am doing. It keeps my fighting skills alive in my mind and it makes the whole world my dojo.

I read a magazine article in which the author, a psychologist, said that when men meet each other for the first time, they consciously or unconsciously size each other up to see if the other is a physical threat to them. According to the doctor, men wonder, however fleetingly, "Can I take this guy?" Well, if that is true, and I think that sometimes it is, the following exercises give you the opportunity to "take this guy" in your imagination.

An innocent guy in a parking lot   You are sitting in your car in a parking lot waiting for someone. Instead of bobbing your head to the newest teenage boy group blasting from your radio, seize the opportunity to observe people. See that big guy walking to his truck over there? Imagine that he is walking toward you. See how he brushes his hair back with his hand? Imagine that he is cocking his fist back to punch you. Visualize your arm shooting out to block it and see yourself snap a slap kick into his groin.

When he reaches his truck, he leans against the tailgate and lights up a cigarette, probably waiting for someone. Note his weight distribution, how he leans his hip against the fender and where both of his hands are. See yourself standing in front of him and exploding forward to foot sweep his closest leg. As he struggles to maintain his balance, follow with a roundhouse kick to his groin, a snapping jab to his throat, and a reverse punch to his chest.

In reality, the poor guy is still leaning against his truck and enjoying his cigarette, unaware you are beating him up.

That loud mouth in line at the movies   You are standing in line at the movies, and while you appear to be patiently tolerating a loud, obnoxious guy in front of you, in your mind you are inflicting some serious mayhem on him. You visualize him starting to push you after you have asked him to please watch his language. You see yourself knock his arm aside and you see your right, roundhouse kick slam into the inside of his closest thigh. You see his head snap forward and you see yourself grab his hair and yank him forward onto his belly.

A guy buying groceries   Look at the guy in front of you at the grocery store checkout stand. Note how he stands with one foot crossed behind his other and how he rests his hand on the counter. Where is his weight? How is he off balance? If you had to dump him, how would you do it given his body position? Imagine taking him the rest of the way off balance and dumping him on the floor. You might just grab him by the back of his collar and pull him over, or you might scoot forward and sweep his foot out from under him. The choice is yours, based on what you think is the best technique for the moment. That is what you are learning with this exercise.

Observe people standing in a variety of positions, so that in time, you are able to take one glance at a person and determine where his balance is weak. Observe how people move, how they distribute their weight when they walk slowly, quickly and even when they run. The more you observe how people move and mentally practice upsetting their balance, the greater the likelihood you will perform well in reality.

Whenever you are on a street corner where there are lots of people, you are literally surrounded by training partners. Have a field day and wade through them punching and kicking as if you were a one-person army. It only takes five seconds, per person, so if you have a 15-minute wait at the bus stop, you can get in lots of reps.

This method of practicing is free of charge, you do not have to give your partner a turn and you get all the target practice and decision making you want.

Imagine Target Selection

In tournament competition, your objective is to punch or kick at legal targets (which are not always the same as vulnerable targets in the street), and if your attack gets in, you earn a point. If it had been a real fight, the blows may have hurt your opponent, maybe not, but as long as you got the flags, you are a happy camper. The street, however, is a different world.

To end a fight quickly in a self-defense situation, your blows must deliver pain and debilitation, and to accomplish that you must strike select vulnerable targets. I encourage you to research information on the best places to hit and to think about which techniques, which strategies and which fighting principles are applicable to a given target or set of targets. Here is a quick list of favorites that have worked for me:

Important

- **Head:** eyes, ears, nose, neck
- **Upper body:** clavicle, sternum, heart, solar plexus, ribs, floating ribs
- **Arms:** biceps, triceps, upper forearm, either side of wrists, back of hands, fingers
- **Lower body:** groin, tail bone, buttocks
- **Legs:** outside thigh, inside thigh, knee area, shin, calf
- **Feet:** Archille's tendon, top of feet, toes

As you watch people on the street and in the malls, observe all their vulnerable targets that are just hanging out and available for hitting. If you had to fight that man walking toward you, which target would you hit first? As he leans against the light pole, what would you hit first to weaken and distract him so that you could hit more vulnerable targets? Consider that clerk handing you your change: Imagine backfisting the fine bones of her fingers, reverse punching her biceps and palm-heeling her nose.

It only takes a fraction of a second to imagine the scenario, and every time you do, you ingrain the concept of target selection in your subconscious

BE ERNEST HEMINGWAY

In *Fighter's Fact Book*, I suggested that you and your training partner take turns "teaching" each other a technique or a combination. Even when both of you are familiar with a movement, the value of this exercise is to articulate the mechanics from beginning to end and do so as specifically as you are able. Verbalizing a move forces you to mentally visualize, analyze and break down every phase of it. In so doing, you develop a greater understanding and clarity of everything that makes it work. Here is a variation on the concept, a form of mental imagery that you do with pen and paper or, if you are a high-tech person, do it on your PC.

Write or type out the way an individual technique or combination is executed. Your imaginary reader is someone who has never seen the movement and therefore needs your explanation to be clear and detailed. Don't leave anything out. Be sure to include how he needs to place his feet when doing his lunge, how he should rotate his hips, how he tucks his chin, how he needs to hold his hands, how he should retract his opposing arm, and so on.

Although I'm familiar with the techniques, drills and exercises discussed in this book, in the process of writing it, I have had to get up repeatedly from my desk and execute the moves in front of a mirror to ensure that I am correctly describing the important elements and that I have included all the necessary details. You should do that, too. Get up, snap out a backfist and check yourself by looking down at your body or at your reflection in a mirror to ensure that you have included everything that needs to be in your written explanation.

I can hear you saying, "But I'm not a writer." Good, I don't need the competition. But I encourage you to do it anyway because it does not matter that you are not Ernest Hemingway. The importance is in the doing, the writing. You can even throw it away when you have finished, since you have already benefitted from the exercise by going through the process. The act of looking at yourself in the mirror, feeling what is going on with your body when you do the technique, and then describing it clearly in your writing, ingrains the intricacies of it in your mind. And you don't even get sweaty.

YOUR INNER TAPES

Did you know that you have invisible audio tapes in your head? If you had good parents, good teachers and supportive friends and training partners, what is recorded on them is positive. But if there have been people in your life who have fed you negative data, and you have heard it so often that you accepted it as valid, the playback on those tapes will be negative, too. On the other hand, if you have been fortunate to have positive information recorded on them, the playback will be positive.

What is on those tapes is so important because it determines how you function in your life and in your training. Consciously or unconsciously, you listen to the playback, and you act accordingly. Please read that again: *You act accordingly* to the information on the tapes.

If your tape says that you are terrible at jump kicks—a result of being told that by a bad teacher or an influential classmate—you will never be able to execute beautiful, aerial leaps as long as you listen to the tape. Your leap will take on either the attributes of a flopping chicken or your landing will go *ku-spalt!* along with your ankle bone. This is because you act out what the tapes whisper to your subconscious mind, which in turn direct your actions.

Important

On the flip side, when your tapes are positive ones, your physical actions will reflect that. *I can jump kick with grace and perfection*, your tapes play, so you jump with grace and perfection. *My kick lashes out with speed, power and flawless form, and I land with grace and control* and so you do it in reality. To reiterate, your physical actions follow the dictates of your inner tapes.

If you have not been conscious of all the negativity you have been exposed to over your training career or even before you took your first lesson, you may not be sure what messages are on your tapes. Unless you want to pay for a psychologist to evaluate where your head is, take a look at the following simple exercise and give it a try. I have taught this for years and always enjoy the positive feedback I get from students.

How to use the list:

Say Them Out Loud

First, get comfy in your favorite chair and take a few deep breaths to get as relaxed as you are able without falling asleep. When you are ready, consider the lists of items here that relate to your fighting art. The first one contains general items, and the one below it contains specific ones. Start with the general. As you go through it, repeat each item aloud several times and then think about each item's meaning before advancing to the next one. Once you have gone through the entire General List, spend a few more minutes thinking about the various items on it. When you are ready, move to the Specific List and say each of those items aloud several times, again thinking about the meaning of each one.

Think Them

The next time you do this exercise, proceed through both lists as before but instead of saying the items aloud, say them in your mind and contemplate the meaning of each one. As before, repeat each item (silently in your mind) several times before moving on to the next one.

Write Them

For your next session, write each one down on a piece of paper. Copy them right out of this book, writing each one several times. Don't allow your mind to wander during your writing, but concentrate on the meaning of what you are putting down. Think of the exercises as sending personal letters to your mind.

Repeating the general and specific statements out loud and thinking about them analytically is pretty darn effortless; but writing them down takes a little work: You have to find some paper, dig through your drawer for a pen and then sit down and do it. Unfortunately, many people skip the writing portion, which means they are omitting a powerful training device that taps straight into their subconscious minds.

Many top athletes striving for the Olympics use the writing exercise. They write down such things as "I *will* qualify for the Olympics" and "I *deserve* to represent my country in the Olympics." Then they write down specific training goals that will advance them toward going. I read recently where basketball players at Duke University, long before the championship game, cover their locker room walls with powerful affirmations, such as, "We are the new national champions!"

Make the lists your own   Feel free to change the two lists to whatever specific statements apply to your objectives. If you have identified in your mind one or more other issues you need to make positive, take out those on this list that do not apply to you and insert those that do.

General List

- I am good at karate
- Karate comes easy to me
- I enjoy the training
- I love the challenge of karate
- I am improving each workout
- I learn quickly
- I accept whatever challenge comes my way
- I am a good martial artist
- I will continue to improve
- I can do anything I work hard on
- I am learning at my own pace
- We all learn at a different pace

Specific List

- I am good at forms
- I am good at kicking
- I am good at punching
- I am good at blocking
- I have fast reflexes
- My speed is good and I am getting faster
- My strength is improving
- I like the challenge of sparring
- I am ready for my belt test
- My tournament techniques are sharp
- If I err, I won't act like it

Don't React to Errors

That last statement, "If I err, I won't act like it," is especially important. I used to have a young student who would go ballistic whenever he erred practicing kata. "Oh man!" he would bellow, clenching his fists, looking to the ceiling and stomping his feet angrily. "I really screwed that up." He reacted the same way when he missed a block in sparring or missed with a kick.

"Don't give your error so much credit," I told him at least 50 times. "Stay cool and keep going. The more you react to an error in your kata, the more you plant a flag in that place so that it will continue to plague you in the future. And it's especially bad when you do it when sparring, Are you going to do that in a real fight?"

"Air" Jordan   Master basketball play Michael Jordan knew this and you can see it in videos of his games. Even after he missed five or six shots in a row, there was no indication of his disappointment: no slumped shoulders, no head drooping, no stomping angrily. Champions like Jordan rarely show their disappointment or anger because they know that they must keep their thoughts positive and not be distracted from the task at hand. They know they must stay focused, aggressive and maintain their peak performance.

Doesn't it make sense that if this is true in basketball that it's also true when you are facing someone bent on ripping your face off? Working on imbedding positive statements in your brain will help you maintain a positive attitude and keep you going no matter what happens.

When you backslide   Even after you have included this list exercise in your solo training for a while, there will be the occasional backsliding when a negative thought seeps in. Don't worry, as that is just being human. Because you have worked on this positive exercise, you will be better able to recognize it when it happens and get busy copying over it with a powerful, positive message.

CROSS TRAINING

I mentioned to a friend at dinner last night that I had had a great solo workout a few hours earlier. He shook his head as if trying to comprehend, and asked, "How do you keep motivated year after year? Heck, how do you stay motivated week after week?" Excellent question.

While a beginning student's enthusiasm over this new and exciting thing called karate keeps him hungry and anxious for the next class, the veteran student often has a hard time putting on the workout gear for one more session. I have to admit that I have those times, too. Here I am penning a book on how to train by yourself and how to psyche yourself to do it, and there are times all I want to do is – nothing. Maybe a little TV. But I never yield to the urge, because (in all humility) I'm too clever for that, and after you finish this chapter, you will be clever, too.

Perhaps you are having trouble facing another session of kicking, punching or kata because you have been training hard all week and you are "full," you are mentally burned out and you need a break from karate. There are also those times when you are physically tired and even the motion of combing your hair is exhausting on arms that have thrown hundreds of punches that week. But your ironclad discipline is driving you to train, to do something. Oh, the dilemma. But unlike other dilemmas you face in life, this one has an easy solution, one that is beneficial for you mentally and physically. It's called cross-training.

Cross-training is a hot concept in the new millennium, a device used by top athletes all over the world to spice up their training by working their muscles and cardiovascular system differently than they normally work them. Cross training gives the athletes a break from their regular training sessions and leaves them physically and mentally refreshed.

Let's take a look at two ways you can use this concept. First let's examine how you can refresh yourself by working on material within your fighting art, but by doing things a little differently than you do normally. Then let's look at some things that you can do outside of your fighting art, things that are remote from punching and kicking, but are nonetheless beneficial.

THINGS TO DO WITHIN THE MARTIAL ARTS

Some might argue that it's really not cross-training if you practice another phase of karate in lieu of what you usually do, because it's ... well, it's still karate. Nonetheless, I'm going to call it cross-training because what you are doing is different and, therefore, it accomplishes your objective of "taking a break" mentally and physically from your usual workout sessions. Allow me to show you some ways that I approach cross-training within my art. Duplicate or modify them as you see fit.

I like 30-minute solo sessions. While this may not sound like a lot of time, I train hard every minute so that the workout is an aerobic one, in which I get in lots of quality repetitions. I rarely do hour-long aerobic solo sessions because they don't fit my time allotment. We are a fast-paced society now, and while most people want to have a good workout in their busy schedule, they don't have a lot of time for it. Fast-paced 30-minute solo sessions can easily fit into the schedules of most fighters, giving them a good aerobic

Workout Tip

session and advancing the quality of their techniques at the same time. If you insist on doing more, simply repeat the workout or add a different 30–minute session.

Here are three fun and productive workouts that are probably different than you do normally.

Workout 1: Be a Boxer

Don't feel like doing karate kicks or backfists? Then train like a boxer. If you don't know how, simply watch a few matches on television and imitate what you see. You might even scoot the chairs and tables back in your television room, and shadowbox along with the fighters who are clashing in the ring. You don't have to box like Mike Tyson; the idea here is to have fun. Here is how to do it in your regular workout area.

Warm up Shuffle about in a boxer's stance, fists held high, chin down, your entire body as loose as a rag doll's. Shuffle, dance, scoot forward, backward and sideways, your arms relaxed and moving about your head as you look for openings.
Warmup: 5 minutes

Mirror punching Stand before a mirror and pop out punches like a boxer. Throw head shots and body shots, straight ones and roundhouse style. Toss in a few uppercuts to your opponent's body and neck. Always put your weight behind your blows and be sure to twist your hips and extend your shoulders. Hey, no backfists. Boxing techniques only.
Punching: 5 minutes

Shadowbox This time, do the same thing you did in front of the mirror, but move about the room as if you were boxing an opponent.
Shadowbox: 10 minutes

Bag work   Punch the bag using boxer-type punches. Move all around it, bobbing, weaving, and moving in and out of range. Hit it as hard or as easily as you like.

Bag work: 6 minutes

Sit-up and punch   Sit on the floor and anchor your feet under something. Keep your knees bent and lower your upper body back until it's at 45 degrees. Using your stomach muscles to pull yourself forward, execute a right boxer's punch as you twist to your left, and execute a left punch as you twist to your right.

Sit-up and punch: 4 minutes

Total time: 30 minutes

Workout 2: An Easy-day Workout

This is for one of those days when your head is telling you to train but your body is telling you to take a Caribbean cruise. Just as you so often have to do in other parts of your life—compromise. An easy day is a workout that does not tax your body, though your muscles get loose, your blood flow increases and, when the session is over, you feel mentally satisfied that you did a little something.

Flow to easy-listening music   Find music that is light, fluid and makes you want to drift upon it like a thistle on a warm, summer breeze (poetic, huh?). The idea is to capture the ebb and flow of your music as you go through your techniques in rhythmic slow motion. For example, extend your foot in a slow motion side kick, set it down gently, swat away an imaginary punch and follow with a slow reverse punch. Slow down. Let your hands float in the air like a Hawaiian hula dancer's. *Feel* the music. *Feel* your gentle movements. *Dance* lightly upon the movement. *Drift* on the breeze. *Feel* the rhythm of the combination.

Do this for shadow sparring, repetition practice and kata. Consider doing all three of these for 10 minutes each.

Total time: 30 minutes

Workout 3: Punch/kick/grapple

I particularly like this idea because it combines karate and grappling and really forces me to think "street" as opposed to just thinking about the mechanics of my technique. There are many ways to format karate with grappling in a 30-minute training session, so you should choose one that you particularly like. Remember, you are cross-training, meaning that you are training differently than you normally do, so get creative with your session. Here is one approach:

Grapple   Choose two of your favorite grappling techniques and pantomime them over and over as many times as you can for 10 minutes. Do them in front of a mirror, looking at yourself from various angles to ensure that you are in top form. Do each technique for five minutes, or if one of the two needs extra work, do it for seven minutes and the other one for three.

Grapple: 10 minutes

Grapple/karate   Stay in front of the mirror for this next session. For five minutes, execute the first grappling technique you just did but add a kick or punch. For the next five minutes, do the second grappling technique, also followed by a punch or kick. Choose karate techniques that flow naturally from whatever position you are in after you have concluded your grappling technique. Check yourself in the mirror from different angles to ensure that your form is proper. Move at whatever speed you want.

Grapple/karate: 10 minutes

Shadow sparring using karate and grappling   Move about the room as you do when you spar, but use only techniques from the two combined karate/grappling techniques in the last paragraph. This forces you to work them in positions that are more realistic to a real fight.

Shadow spar: 10 minutes

Total time: 30 minutes

Workout 4: Stations

This is a fun way to train in your regular karate class and it's also fun to do when training alone. If you have access to your regular karate school, set up your stations all around the room. If you have to train in your house or a small apartment, no problem, you can still use the station format. Let's take a look at both situations.

Your school   Since I don't know what equipment you have, let me explain how I set up my room in my school.

Station 1: I begin by shadow sparring in front of my big mirror. I do everything I normally do in a sparring session: punch, kick, block, duck and shuffle. Although, I have done a warm-up, I always make the mirror my first station to ensure that all my joints and other goodies are completely loose and lubricated.
Shadow sparring: 5 minutes

Station 2:   Now it's time to eat some humble pie and move over to the double-end bag. It's not about hitting it hard, but hitting it accurately when it's wobbling all over the place. I move all around it, hitting with the best technique that fits the moment.
Double-end bag: 5 minutes

Station 3:   I choose two stepping movements, such as the lunge and crossover, and I do them as many times as I can in the allotted time. I push for speed and power.
Stepping: 10 minutes

Station 4:   I face the heavy bag and go nuts, holding nothing back as I punch, kick, rip and headbutt. It's survival time, and I'm out to save my bacon.
Heavy bag: 5 minutes

Station 5:   I strap on a bungee cord and do 20 reps each leg of front kick and 10 reps each leg of the side kick.
Bungee cord kicking: 5 minutes

Total Time: 30 minutes

Apartment/House Station Training   This is fun and beneficial since you are training in a real-world environment: your living space.

Station 1: Warm up by shadow sparring in, what is probably your most spacious room, the living area. Don't move anything out of the way, but rather shadow spar around that coffee table and antique China cabinet. (I was working my sickles in my living room one time and accidentally hacked off three feet of a dangling houseplant.)
Shadow sparring: 5 minutes

Station 2:   Go into that narrow hallway that leads from the living room to the back bedrooms and practice kicking. Don't just stand in place and do them, but rather move about so that you are forced to contend with the narrow space. Does leaning against the walls and doorways help your kicking power?
Hallway kicking: 10 minutes

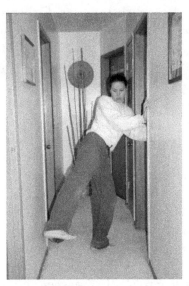

See what you can and cannot do in that narrow hallway in your home.

Station 3:   Now you are off to the bathroom. During my career as a police officer, I fought with people many times in bathrooms, public and private. It's not fun, especially when it's a skid row restroom with overflowing toilets. No matter how small your bathroom, shadow spar in it and deal with the confined space. Learn what techniques you can and cannot do.

Bathroom shadow sparring: 5 minutes

Station 4:   I've also been in several fights in bedrooms (on-duty, thank you), and while not as disgusting as bathrooms, they still offer many challenges. For example, try your punching and kicking reps in that space between the bed and the wall. What kicks can you not do in the confined space? Are there any you can do? Can you still throw a punch when your back is against the wall and you are pinned next to the dresser? If not, what can you do?

Bedroom reps: 10 minutes

Total time: 30 minutes

These ideas for cross-training within your fighting art don't even scratch the surface of what you can do that is different, fun, innovative and productive. The idea is to train within your art differently than you normally do. Here are a few other ideas off the top of my head. Consider all of them 30-minute workouts.

- Do punches, kicks and blocks in a swimming pool
- Run a quarter mile, stop and do one minute of as many kicks and punches as you can. Repeat the run and stop three more times until you have completed a mile.
- Choose one technique and do it standing, sitting, lying on the floor, in bed, on one knee, etc.
- Put on a silly martial arts movie and punch and kick along with the fight scenes.
- Practice fighting techniques inside your car

Keep in mind that your objective when cross training within your art is to train differently than you normally do.

NON-MARTIAL ARTS ACTIVITIES

Black Belt Hall of Fame member Ernie Reyes Sr. has had a long competitive career and is well known for his West Coast Demo Team's incredible display of martial arts excellence. He credits cross-training for giving him a competitive edge in his early years and for later enhancing his quality of life in his still-active martial arts career. While he uses other fighting arts for cross-training within his art, such as Tae-bo, Muay Thai kickboxing and jujitsu, he also enjoys cross-training in esoteric activities that at first glance may not seem applicable.

Gardening   "Gardening—as unrelated as it may seem from kicking, punching and the West Coast Demo Team—has taught me a better sense of the natural order of things," Reyes said in *Martial Arts Training*, January 2000 issue. "It may sound like a cliche', but having a garden teaches you about patience and nurturing … qualities that will help any instructor. Gardening also gets me closer to nature. It's like a soothing meditation."

If a champion like Reyes benefits from cross-training in his garden, the door is wide open as to what you can do (no, channel surfing doesn't count). Let's look at typical cross-training ideas that I have stolen from other karate people. All of these work your muscles, though differently than your regular karate training. As we did in "Things to do within your art," the following are done in 30-minute sessions. Of course, you can increase the time if you want.

Yoga	Aerobic dance class
Jogging	Stretching
Sprinting	Swimming
Circuit training with weights	Bicycling
Military calisthenics	Baseball
Tennis	Jumping rope
Fast walking	Hiking

For some fighters, their aerobic condition is activity specific, meaning, they can spar for 30 minutes but jog for only 15, or vice versa. If this is you, use cross-training to round out your fitness. Make sure you are getting aerobic conditioning in your karate, but also make sure you are in shape to run, swim, bicycle and do any of the other activities on the list that interest you. Be sure to include rest days in between so that you don't get burnt out.

Caution

Below are a few activities that are more meditative than those listed above. You may not work up a big sweat with these, but your fighting art will still benefit as your muscles rest and your brain "gets some air" from your usual training regimen. Some of the following directly impact your progress, while others help you get in touch with your inner self.

- Meditate
- Visualize
- Read a book on psychology or philosophy
- Hike in the wilderness
- Listen to inspirational music
- Go fishing
- Go camping
- Lay under a tree

Practice visualizing your techniques for an easy, sweatless but productive workout.

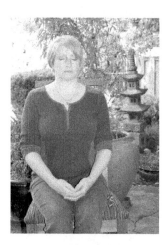

Putting it All Together

No matter how long you have trained, you will benefit from cross-training. Use it to completely change your solo workout from what you normally do, or do part of your regular karate workout for 15 minutes, and then do something outside of your fighting art for the remaining 15. It's your solo time, time that you don't have to answer to anyone. Do it your way. If you normally train in a space in your basement, train in your living room the next time. If you are on a business trip, train in your hotel room, take a 30-minute swim in the pool or, if they have a workout room, hit the stationary bike for 30 minutes. Maybe the hotel offers an aerobic class or the front desk can direct you to one close by. Once I participated in a hotel's aerobic class. The ab routine, which was completely different and tougher than even the 300-count one we do in my school, left me nearly gasping on the floor in the fetal position. Once the soreness went away, I looked back on it as fun. Sorta.

Broaden your horizons   Cross training puts spark into your training, which is especially important during those periods when you are getting bored or burnt out from doing the same thing time after time. It refreshes your body and it refreshes your mind. It's also about keeping you physically and mentally balanced. Instead of just being a guy who converses only on karate, cross-training educates you about other activities. You are able to talk to your running friends about running and your weight lifting friends about lifting. A nice side benefit to broadening your horizons is that you will discover elements in these activities that help you learn more about yourself.

Study of the martial arts is a journey of self-discovery, but you can use other paths to help you along the way. Experiment with cross-training and discover more of what you are about.

12 WORKOUTS

Here are twelve 30-minute solo workouts that I have used for years. Some of them are easy and some are real energy drainers. If you sit down for an hour with pen and paper and this book, you could easily come up with 30 more. If you researched for an entire afternoon, you could come up with dozens of workouts. Consider the ones I have provided here as just a starting point, a base that you can add to and subtract from. Since real fights are extraordinarily taxing, I always do my solo training aerobically, and I encourage you to do them the same.

I usually train alone on Saturday mornings. I go nuts for 30 minutes and even though I usually feel like doing more, I force myself to stop. I stretch for 10 minutes and then hit the shower. Afterwards, I feel energized, loose and ready to enjoy the day.

Hour-long sessions test your mettle and your endurance. Many fighters like the longer sessions because they can work on more material and because they feel that they just don't get enough with the shorter ones. If this is you that is okay. But understand that just because you prefer the hour workouts, it does not mean that the shorter ones are not good for you, too. They are. If you like the longer ones, fine. But if time and lack of energy forces you to do a 30-minute one, don't feel guilty. You will benefit from the 30-minute session and, if you train correctly, you will even make progress.

Admittedly, I'm getting older, but that is not what is influencing my advocacy of short, intense workouts. In my 20s I often trained with several guys from 9:00am to 5pm. Was the training nonstop? No. Anyone who tells you they train nonstop that long is fibbing or fooling themselves. When I had those all-day sessions, we trained, chatted, trained some more, stretched, trained some more, chatted and so on. Although there were lots of down times, our young bodies still suffered from chronic fatigue, injuries, illness and burnout.

Training Tip

I was to realize years later, about the same time that tons of supporting literature came out, that more is not better when it comes to training. Experts in the field of fitness and training now advocate shorter, more intense workouts as opposed to lengthy, less intense ones. Without going into a long explanation of all the physiological reasons why short workouts are good for you, just know that they prevent overtraining, they help maintain your enthusiasm (on low motivation days, it's easier to convince yourself to do a 30-minute session than a 60-minute one) and, something that is important in this fast-paced world, short, hard workouts save you precious time. Go ahead and do those long workouts when you want to, but keep in mind that the short ones are good, too.

DETERMINING YOUR HEART RATE

When exercising aerobically, you want to raise your pulse rate to between 60 and 90 percent of your maximum heart rate. If you are in great shape aerobically and experienced with aerobic exercise, train at 85 percent with occasional jumps into the 90 percent range. If you are out of shape, you should train at 60 percent, increasing to 65 percent in about two weeks and to 75 two weeks after that. If progressing every two weeks is too fast for you, then make it three weeks, or four. If you are consistent in your training, progress in your aerobic fitness will come faster than can imagine. As always, you are advised to check with a physician before beginning any strenuous exercise program.

You can find your pulse on the side of your neck or on your wrist below the base of your thumb. During your workout, check your pulse at least twice. Count your heartbeats for 6 seconds and multiply the number by 10 to determine your heart rate per minute. If it's ticking too slow, increase the intensity of your training; if it's too high, slow things down a little.

Here is an easy way to determine your heart rate when exercising aerobically. Begin with a base number of 220 for males, 226 for females and subtract your age. Let's say you are a 20-year-old male in fair aerobic condition and you want to train at 75 percent of your maximum heart rate.

$$
\begin{array}{rl}
& 220 \quad \text{male (226 female)} \\
\text{Subtract:} & \underline{20} \quad \text{age} \\
& 200 \quad \text{maximum heart rate} \\
\text{Multiply:} & \underline{.75} \quad \text{percent of maximum heart rate} \\
\text{Total:} & 150 \quad \text{beats per minute}
\end{array}
$$

This means that you will elevate your heart rate to 150 beats per minute for the entire 30-minute workout.

The old school of thought on aerobic training was that you could not stop during the exercise because your heart rate would recover and, therefore negate the training effect of the aerobic exercise. Fitness experts no longer believe that stopping is detrimental. In fact, some say that you can split your session. For example, do 15 minutes in the morning and 15 in the afternoon.

On the following pages are the 12, 30-minute workouts. Let's begin with the only one that is not aerobic.

Light Stretch Workout

You can also call this the "Feel-Good Stretch Workout" because, well, it just feels good. Do it on days when you are not in class, as a way to relax after you have gotten home from your regular karate class, after a stressful day at work or school, or when you just want to feel a burst of energy.

Half way through writing this book, I took a week-long vacation and did the Easy Stretch Workout every day. Since I promised myself that I would let my body rest and recuperate from the weights and martial arts, I stretched as a way to wind down from walking around all those tourist traps and as a way to get loose on those days I did nothing except eat. The workout left me refreshed and energized and –surprise, surprise – it even increased my flexibility. I wasn't trying to increase it, but because I did the routine every day, I progressed beyond what had been my maximum stretch.

Although you don't push the stretches, it's still important to first warm up the muscles. Do 10 reps with each leg of straight-leg lifts to the front to loosen your hips and hamstrings, 10 reps with each straight leg to the side to loosen the hips and groin muscles, 10 straight-leg lifts to the rear to warm up the ol' butt muscles and 10 roundhouse chambers with each leg to loosen your hips a tad more.

It doesn't matter when you stretch or where, as long as you just do it. Stretching is a no brainer, so you can easily do other things while you sink into the pose. Television time is a perfect opportunity because all you have to do is plop yourself down on the floor or stretch your leg out on the back of a chair and begin stretching. Consider spreading the newspaper out in front of you and catch up on the news. Bruce Lee used to hold a stretch, read a book and do dumbbell curls all at the same time.

I like to rest my foot on my balcony rail and read a magazine as I hold my pose for one minute, switch legs and do another minute, continuing in this fashion for 10-15 minutes. Then I drop down on the floor, spread 'em with the magazine between my legs, and do a few more minutes.

The specific stretches are for you to choose. You can push yourself to increase your flexibility if you want, but the basic idea with the East Stretch Workout is to loosen your muscles and release energy into them. If you take this easy approach, you might happily discover that your flexibility will begin increasing, seemingly without effort. It's true that sometimes when you quit trying so hard at something, in this case stretching, and just do the activity for the enjoyment, you suddenly start progressing. I've seen it happen with people trying to make gains in their weight training and people training in the martial arts. So just mellow out, dude. Relax and enjoy the feeling.

How long you hold each stretch posture is up to you, as there doesn't seem to be an agreement among experts as to the length of time. Some say 15 seconds, other experts say 60, while still others claim that 5-minute postures are best. I advise 30-60 seconds. One incredibly flexible gymnast friend agreed, and said, "You should hold each stretch for 30-60 seconds, and hold it right on the edge of the pain. If you want to improve your static flexibility, you should stretch seven times a week, at least once per day for 20 minutes each session. If you want to just maintain your current level, two to four times a week will do it."

Light Stretch Workout

Time: 30 minutes

WARM UP

Straight-leg lifts to the front
    2 sets, 10 reps
    both legs
Straight-leg lifts to the side
    2 sets, 10 reps
    both legs
Straight-leg lifts to the rear
    2 sets, 10 reps
    both legs
Roundhouse chambers
    2 sets, 10 reps
    both legs

STRETCHES

One or two exercises for the back of your legs (hamstrings)
    1 set, 5 reps
    both legs (hold for 30-60 seconds)
One or two exercises for the inside of your legs (groin muscles)
    1 set, 5 reps
    both legs (hold 30-60 seconds)
One or two exercises for your hips (Leg Chambering)
    1 set, 5 reps
    both legs hold (10-30 seconds)

TIP

When warming up with the straight leg kicks and chambering, lift your legs at medium speed and as high as you can. The keyword in this session is "easy." Don't sweat and strain; you are doing this just to feel good and to energize yourself. Repeat any or all exercises until you have stretched for 30 minutes.

WORKOUT NOTES:

Boxer-Type Workout

I call this a boxer-*type* workout because it's typical of how boxers train by themselves using the three-minute round system. If you are out of condition, begin with three, three-minute rounds and progressively add a round as your wind improves, until you are doing 10, three-minute rounds. Doing all of the rounds takes 40 minutes, counting the one minute rest period in between each round. When you get to this point, you will be in fantastic condition, a lean, mean fighting machine.

The format is simple: You go all out for three minutes, rest for one minute and then do another three minutes. Be sure to work both sides when applicable.

Boxer-Type Workout

Time: 40 minutes

Round 1:
    Side-straddle hops (1 minute)
    Fast abdominal crunches (2 minutes)

Rest 1 minute

Round 2:
    Footwork: move around as if you were facing
        an opponent (2 minutes)
    Fast abdominal crunches (1 minute)

Rest 1 minute

Round 3:
    Jabs with footwork (1 minute)
    Backfists with footwork (1 minute)
    Fast abdominal crunches (1 minute)

Rest 1 minute

Round 4:
    Reverse punches (2 minutes)
    Footwork (1 minute)

Rest 1 minute

Round 5:
    Jab, reverse punch combination (1 minute)
    Knee strike (1 minute)

Rest 1 minute

Round six:
    Front kicks (1 minute)
    Roundhouse kicks (1 minute)
    Side kicks (1 minute)

Rest 1 minute

Round 7:
    Backfists, roundhouse kicks (1 minute)
    Front kicks, jabs (2 minutes)

Rest 1 minute

Round 8:
    Side kicks, turning back kicks (2 minutes)
    Double roundhouse kicks (1 minute)

Rest 1 minute

Round 9:
    Shadow spar (3 minutes)

Rest 1 minute

Round 10:
    Shadow spar (3 minutes)

Collapse

TIP

Use this 10-round workout as is, or modify it as you see fit. Consider doing some of the rounds on the bag and some in the air. Your goal, and it's an admirable one, is to go through all 10 rounds as hard and fast as you are able. Take a swig of water during your one-minute rest and breathe in deeply through your nose, so that your lower abdomen expands, and exhale slowly out of your mouth. Water and fresh oxygen are your only friends during this killer workout.

WORKOUT NOTES:

Heavy Bag Workout: Hands Only

The primary concern while working the heavy bag (besides not spraining your joints) is to ensure that your heart rate doesn't get too high, which is easy to do on the bag because you are having such a good time wailing on it. But if after 10 minutes you find that your heart is beating at 90 percent of your maxim heart rate and you don't want to go that high, you need to reduce the intensity of your blows. You can do that by backing away from the bag and doing a little light air punching until your heart rate lowers somewhere between 75-85 percent.

Keep in mind that you don't have to throw every technique all out. One way to determine how hard you are hitting is by using this simple measuring device.

Level 1: Light to medium
Level 2: Hard

Mix up the levels as you work the bag. Do three minutes of Level 1 and then one minute at Level 2. Then do five minutes at Level 1 and five minutes at Level 2.

Okay, let's do some slugging. Assume your fighting stance and begin shuffling around the bag as if sparring with a partner.

<u>WORKOUT NOTES:</u>

Heavy Bag Workout: Hands Only

Time: 30 minutes

Reverse punch with lunge step
    1 set, 15 reps
    both sides
Roundhouse palm-heel strike with lunge step
    1 set, 15 reps
    both sides
U punch with lunge step
    1 set, 10 reps
    both sides
Backfist with crossover step
    1 set, 15 reps
    both sides
Backfist and reverse punch
    1 set, 10 reps
    both sides
Chair punching jab/reverse punch combination:
    1 set, 10 reps
    both sides
Random hitting
    3 minutes at Level 1
Random hitting
    1 minute at Level 2

TIP

When doing "Chair punching," position your chair one or two steps from the bag, and then spring out of it, lunge and hit. If you get through the entire list in 10 minutes, repeat two more times for a 30-minute, heavy bag workout.

Heavy Bag Workout: Legs Only

Allow me to be your mother for a moment. Having had the not-so-fun experience of blowing a kneecap 10 years into my martial arts training, I realized early on the importance of that fragile joint. Although sore knees are part of the martial arts, any time yours hurts, whether it's just for three days or three months, do not kick the bag. Let your knee heal first. Period. No exceptions. Okay, let's move on.

Assume your fighting stance and begin shuffling around the bag as if sparring with a partner, and proceed through the following list.

WORKOUT NOTES:

Heavy Bag Workout: Legs Only

Time: 30 minutes

Angle front kick with a replacement step
    1 set 15 reps
    both sides
Roundhouse shin kick with a replacement step
    1 set, 15 reps
    both sides
Funny kick, no step
    1 set, 15 reps
    both sides
Side kick (tight chamber) with a replacement
step   1 set, 15 reps
    both sides
Rear leg crescent with a slide step
    1 set, 10 reps
    both sides
Touch back kick, no step
    1 set, 10 reps
    both sides

TIP

Although low licks are the most effective in a self-defense situation, kick the bag at various heights so that your leg muscles get a well-rounded workout. If you get through all of the exercises in 10 minutes, work through the list two more times for a 30-minute heavy bag workout.

Heavy Bag: Elbows and Knees

Whether your heavy bag is a hanging one or a freestanding manikin type, this drill requires that you virtually position yourself chest-to-bag as you rain elbows and knees on it.

WORKOUT NOTES:

Heavy Bag: Elbows and Knees

Time: 30 minutes

Inside knee strike
 1 set, 15 reps
 both sides
Round knee, rear leg
 1 set 15 reps
 both sides
Round knee, front leg
 1 set, 15 reps
 both sides
Horizontal elbow
 1 set, 15 reps
 both sides
Round elbow
 1 set, 15 reps
 both sides
Downward round elbow
 1 set, 15 reps
 both sides
Random elbows and knees
 2 minutes

TIP

Since elbowing and kneeing the bag is especially strenuous on your hips and shoulders, be sure to thoroughly warm them up first. If you get through the entire list in 10 minutes, repeat two more times for a 30-minute heavy bag workout.

Shadow Spar and Crunches

Combining shadow sparring and abdominal crunches in a 30-minute a solo training session works virtually every muscle in your body. The sporadic abdominal work gives you a moment of rest (not much) from your kicking and punching and, when the session is over, leaves your midsection feeling nice and tight. Put on your favorite tunes or train to silence. You can shadow spar using any techniques that come to mind, or you can use your session to incorporate material from this book, say, one or two techniques from each section. If you just want to emphasize your hands, pick one or more hand techniques to work on, or select a couple of kicks if you want to just work your legs. It's your choice because it's your workout.

As you spar, watch the clock. Every five minutes, drop to the floor and knock out one or two sets of an abdominal crunch exercise of your choice. When you have completed them, jump back to your feet and get sparring again.

WOKROUT NOTES:

Shadow Spar and Crunches

Time: 30 minutes

Shadow spar
   6 minutes
Abdominal crunches
   2 minutes
Shadow spar
   6 minutes
Abdominal crunches
   2 minutes
Shadow spar
   6 minutes
Abdominal crunches
   2 minutes
Shadow spar
   6 minutes

TIP

Change your level of intensity as you spar. For example, do one six-minute sparring session at Level 1 and the next at Level 2, and so on. Get up and down from the floor as quickly as you can and always rep out your abdominal crunches with good form.

Body Work Cardio Workout

As the name implies, this entire workout is done without throwing one little ol' punch or kick. It's a good aerobic session for those days you want to train, but your arms and legs are tired or your elbow and knee joints are crying for a day off.

<u>WORKOUT NOTES:</u>

Body Work Cardio Workout

Time: 30 minutes

Mirror slipping
    5 minutes
Abdominal crunches
    5 minutes
Foot work
    5 minutes
Abdominal crunches
    5 minutes
Mirror slipping
    5 minutes
Getting up from the floor
    5 minutes

TIP

Fluctuate your speed of execution in each 5-minute block. When doing, say, Mirror slipping, do one minute at Level 1 and then one minute at Level 2 and then one minute at Level 1 again. Continue in this fashion through all the exercises. If you are in great shape and want a tough workout, perform every minute at top speed.

Cross Training

You want to work on your punches and kicks, but you don't want to do 30 minutes of them. Try breaking up the session with 15 minutes of cross training outside your fighting art and 15 minutes of cross training inside your fighting art.

WORKOUT NOTES:

Cross Training

Cross Training Within you Art

Shadow spar (hands only) in your bathroom
    5 minutes

Kicking reps in your cluttered garage or basement
    front kicks (1 minute)
    roundhouse kicks (1 minute)
    side kicks (1 minute)
    back kicks (1 minute)
    knee strikes (1 minute)
                Total: 5minutes

Shadow spar in your hallway
    5 minutes

Cross Train Outside your Art

Fast walk or jog outside
    15 minutes

TIP

This is a great way to train when on vacation or a business trip. Train within your art in your hotel room – in the bathroom, between the bed and the wall, in the entryway – and then train 15 minutes outside your art by jogging, swimming hard laps in the hotel swimming pool or using their workout facility to do stationary bicycle or circuit training with weights. Get creative with what is available.

Resistance Punching/Cardio

This routine gives you a nice mix of exercises to build power in your hand techniques the first half of the session, and then multiple kicks the last half to get your heart and lungs really burning. Although weight resistance exercises are never done fast, you still get a mild aerobic workout when you do them with only 15-30-second rest periods between sets. When all the hand techniques have been completed, use whatever time is left for kicking.

WORKOUT NOTES:

Resistance Punching/Cardio

Time: 30 minutes

Jab with dumbbells
    3 sets, 10 reps
    both sides
Reverse punch with dumbbells
    3 sets, 10 reps
    both sides
Backfist with bungee cord
    3 sets, 10 reps
    both sides
Roundhouse punch
    3 sets, 10 reps
    both sides
Choose one, two or three kicks and do them hard and fast in the time remaining. For example: Alternate front kicks (1 minute) with hook kicks (1 minute) until your 30-minute session is over.

TIP

One variation is to do one minute of kicks between each completed punching exercise. For example, do 3 sets of 10 reps with "Jab with dumbbells," and then one minute of fast kicks. When finished, proceed to "Reverse punch with dumbbells." When you have finished all of the hand exercises with the one minute of interspersed kicking, use the time left to do more kicks.

Ground Techniques

This is a real energy drainer, one that will get you breathing like an old workhorse. You simply lie down on the ground and then scramble to your feet, preferably using one of the methods described in this book. When you are all the way up, drop back down (if you know how to fall, drop with a slapout) and repeat the procedure.

TIP

If you are out of shape, do the reps slowly at first, concentrating on good form (you will still get a mild aerobic workout). As your conditioning improves over the weeks, pick up the pace. When you are in top shape aerobically, push to get as many reps in as you can in each session while maintaining good form. The instant you have gotten to your feet, drop back down to the floor.

WORKOUT NOTES:

Ground Techniques

Time: 30 minutes

Drop to the floor & get up as quickly as you can
    Alternate side and runner's position
    5 minutes

Drop down on your back, continue fighting as
you get up
    5 minutes

Drop onto your stomach and, as you scramble to
your feet, slip one or two of your imaginary
attacker's punches and kicks
    5 minutes

Get down on your hands and knees. Alternate
10 reps of roundhouse chambers with 10 reps of
sidekick chambers
    5 minutes

Drop onto your back, and continue fighting as
you get up, incorporate one or two blocks against
imaginary punches and kicks
    5 minutes

Drop onto your stomach and get up as quickly as
you can (repeat of the first exercise)
    5 minutes

Air/Bag Drill

Begin by punching the heavy bag for 15 minutes and then punching the air for 15. The bag will help you develop hand power and punching the air will help you develop speed. You can eventually insert any hand techniques you want, but to start out, humor me and use these often-ignored techniques that have been discussed in this book.

TIP

Notice that the techniques for the bag and those for air striking are the same. One variation is to alternate hitting the bag and the air. For example, do the hammer strike for three minutes on the bag and then the hammer strike for three minutes in the air. Continue alternating bag, air, bag, air until you have completed all of the hand techniques.

WORKOUT NOTES:

Air/Bag Drill

Time: 30 minutes

Heavy Bag

> Hammer strike, both sides, your choice of angle
> > 3 minutes
>
> Slap strike, both sides, your choice of angle
> > 3 minutes
>
> Knife hand thrust, both sides
> > 3 minutes
>
> Forearm strike, both sides, your choice of angle
> > 3 minutes
>
> U punch, both sides
> > 3 minutes

Total: 15 minutes

Air

> Hammer strike, both sides, your choice of angle
> > 3 minutes
>
> Slap strike, both sides, your choice of angle
> > 3 minutes
>
> Knife hand thrust, both sides
> > 5 minutes
>
> Forearm strike, both sides, your choice of angle
> > 3 minutes
>
> U punch, both sides
> > 3 minutes

Total: 15 minutes

Kata and Kata Breakdown

There are two parts to this 30-minute session. In one, you do a kata as many times as you can in 15 minutes. If your kata takes two minutes, you can squeeze in six, maybe seven run throughs, allowing for a few second to catch your breath in between. The last half of your workout is spent drilling on one or two sequences from your kata that you want to give extra attention. A sequence may have two techniques, or as many as five.

WORKOUT TIPS:

Kata and Kata Breakdown

Time: 30 minutes

Kata in its entirety
  5-7 times with a 30-second rest period
  15 minutes

One or two sequences, performed repetitiously
  15 minutes

TIP

Perform both 15-minute blocks hard, fast and with as much mental intensity as you can. Believe that you are in a real fight and you will perform accordingly.

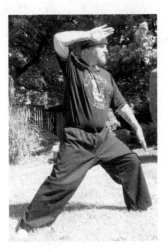

This classic kata move is unrealistic for real combat. How can it be modified to be applicable for the street?

CONCLUSION

So, have I convinced you to incorporate solo training into your martial arts studies? If not, please try this experiment for three months. It costs you only one hour a week of television and, since you do only one 30-minute session at a time, you miss only two, half-hour programs. Here is the experiment.

Attend your martial arts classes as you normally do, but add one 30-minute training session twice a week for three months. What you do during these sessions is up to you, but as long as you are devoting time to it, strive to progress in an area in which you feel you need improvement, especially an area that gets little attention in your classes. Or, consider working on something that is new to you, something you learned in this book, or something you picked up elsewhere.

Do you want to be more aerobically fit for your fighting art? Do you want faster and stronger kicks? Hand techniques that hit as fast as a mad drummer's? Or do you want to learn a couple of new techniques and see how far you can progress with them in three months?

Whatever you choose to do, use this book to plan your attack. Read the description of each technique, drill and exercise that you want to incorporate into your training to ensure that you are doing them properly. Begin your three-month training period using the sets and reps I have recommended herein. After the first two workouts, ask yourself if you need to reduce or increase them. Continue to evaluate yourself and the workout every two weeks for the entire three months.

So, what can you expect for your one hour a week investment? Take it from a guy who has been supplementing his training with solo workouts since 1965, and who has been teaching others to do the same for nearly as many years: If you train consistently and intelligently, you, as well as others, will see marked progress from where you began three months earlier.

Not a bad deal for a one-hour investment out of your entire week, and that was just after incorporating training alone for three months. If you make training alone part of your life, just imagine where you will be in six months. In one year. And it only takes an hour a week.

It does not get much better than that.

Do it.

Acknowledgments

Many thanks to the photographers:
Amy S. Christensen
Donna-Duff Christensen
Laura Whited

and to the models:
Alain Burrese
Donna-Duff Christensen
Amy S. Christensen
Dan L. Christenesen
Professor Tim Delgman
Manny Polanco
Mark Whited
Tim Sukimoto
The old guy is me

and to the martial arts experts who shared their knowledge:

Instructor Marc "Animal" MacYoung has worked as a body-guard, bouncer, event security provider and director of a correctional institute. As he says, "I'm a man, who despite the best efforts of his enemies, is still breathing." He has taken that experience and his eclectic martial arts experience and written several books and made numerous videos on the fighting arts. Check out his site at:
No Nonsense Self-defense Web Page
http://www.diac.com/~dgordon/index.html

Instructor Daniel Alix, currently a captain in the United States Army, has been training and teaching tang soo do for 20 years. He has also studied karate, taekwondo and hapkido and slants his teaching toward street defense. He is currently stationed on the West Coast.

Instructor **Bob Orlando** has studied aikido, iaido, arnis, and eskrima. However, what has impacted the most is the years he has studied Chinese kuntao and Indonesian pentjak silat under Dutch-Indonesian master William de Thouars. He still studies with the master today and resides in Colorado. Check out his site at *Je Doo-Tu School of Martial Arts* http://www.OrlandoKuntao.com

Instructor **Frank Garza** has been studying American Kenpo Karate for many years and is a ranking black belt under Sifu Rick Fowler. He has also studied, judo, muay Thai, silat, kali and jujitsu. He resides in Texas.

Instructor **Alain Burrese** is a former infantry paratrooper with the 82nd Airborne Division and scout sniper with the 2nd Infantry Division in South Korea. He has studied a variety of martial arts and while in Korea earned high ranking from the Korea Hapkido Federation. Check out his site at *The Tao of Warriorship* http://members.aol.com/aburrese/

Instructor **Steve Golden's** formal martial arts training began in 1959 when he began studying kenpo karate under Ed Parker. In 1965, he began teaching keno. Steve first met Bruce Lee in 1964 at Ed Parker's school in Pasadena, California. Steve started training at Bruce's school in Los Angles the day it opened in 1967 and was also a member of the group who trained at Bruce's home. He teaches a group of students in Oregon and Washington and gives national and international seminars.

Instructor **Richard Kirkham** has been studying the martial arts for 28 years. He is a dual certified teacher with a Bachelors of Science Degree in Physical Education with a background in special education, exercise physiology, movement education, and behavioral modification. He is presently an in-home tutor, self-defense instructor, and bodyguard. Richard is presently teaching in Honolulu Hawaii. Check out his *Martial Arts Ezine* at http://tutor.hypermart.net/martialarts_ezine.html

Instructor David J. Bean is a veteran martial artist who focuses his studies on karate and jujitsu.

Steve Perry is a well-known freelance science fiction writer with over 40 books to his credit, as well TV scripts, short stories, assorted non-fiction articles and movie scripts. His previous experience as a physician's assistance was helpful when I needed questions answered about the implications of karate blows. He has studied several martial arts systems and is currently studying the Indonesian martial art of pentjak silat. Check out his site at *Welcome to Steve Perry's Web Page* http://www.teleport.com/~sperry/Index.html

Instructor Kenneth A. Smith has spent over 30 years as a student and practitioner of the martial arts and various mystical disciplines of the world. He is versed in more than 50 different systems from 17 different countries. He gives much credit to his instructor, Fong Su-Yi, creator of Tai-Yang Lung Tao. Check out his web site at *The Way of the Sun Dragon* http://sundragon.easternjewels.com/

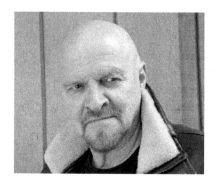

ABOUT THE AUTHOR

Loren W. Christensen is a Vietnam veteran and retired police officer with 29 years of law enforcement experience.

As a martial arts student and teacher since 1965, he has earned an 8th dan in American Free Style Karate, a 2nd dan in aiki jujitsu, and a 1st dan in Modern Arnis. He has starred in seven instructional martial arts DVDs. In 2011, Loren was inducted into the Masters Hall of Fame, garnering the Golden Lifetime Achievement Award.

As a writer, Loren has worked with five publishers, penning over 50 books, nonfiction and fiction on a variety of subjects. His thriller fiction series *Dukkha* is popular among martial artists. He has written dozens of magazine articles on a variety of topics to include, martial arts, nutrition, bodybuilding, police tactics, survival skills, meditation, and mental imagery.

He can be contacted through his website at www.lwcbooks.com.

Index

BOOKS FROM YMAA

6 HEALING MOVEMENTS
101 REFLECTIONS ON TAI CHI CHUAN
108 INSIGHTS INTO TAI CHI CHUAN
ADVANCING IN TAE KWON DO
ANALYSIS OF SHAOLIN CHIN NA 2ND ED
ANCIENT CHINESE WEAPONS
ART OF HOJO UNDO
ARTHRITIS RELIEF, 3RD ED.
BACK PAIN RELIEF, 2ND ED.
BAGUAZHANG, 2ND ED.
CARDIO KICKBOXING ELITE
CHIN NA IN GROUND FIGHTING
CHINESE FAST WRESTLING
CHINESE FITNESS
CHINESE TUI NA MASSAGE
CHOJUN
COMPREHENSIVE APPLICATIONS OF SHAOLIN
    CHIN NA
CONFLICT COMMUNICATION
CROCODILE AND THE CRANE: A NOVEL
CUTTING SEASON: A XENON PEARL MARTIAL ARTS
    THRILLER
DEFENSIVE TACTICS
DESHI: A CONNOR BURKE MARTIAL ARTS THRILLER
DIRTY GROUND
DR. WU'S HEAD MASSAGE
DUKKHA HUNGRY GHOSTS
DUKKHA REVERB
DUKKHA, THE SUFFERING: AN EYE FOR AN EYE
DUKKHA UNLOADED
ENZAN: THE FAR MOUNTAIN, A CONNOR BURKE MARTIAL
    ARTS THRILLER
ESSENCE OF SHAOLIN WHITE CRANE
EXPLORING TAI CHI
FACING VIOLENCE
FIGHT BACK
FIGHT LIKE A PHYSICIST
THE FIGHTER'S BODY
FIGHTER'S FACT BOOK
FIGHTER'S FACT BOOK 2
FIGHTING THE PAIN RESISTANT ATTACKER
FIRST DEFENSE
FORCE DECISIONS: A CITIZENS GUIDE
FOX BORROWS THE TIGER'S AWE
INSIDE TAI CHI
KAGE: THE SHADOW, A CONNOR BURKE MARTIAL ARTS
    THRILLER
KATA AND THE TRANSMISSION OF KNOWLEDGE
KRAV MAGA PROFESSIONAL TACTICS
KRAV MAGA WEAPON DEFENSES
LITTLE BLACK BOOK OF VIOLENCE
LIUHEBAFA FIVE CHARACTER SECRETS
MARTIAL ARTS ATHLETE
MARTIAL ARTS INSTRUCTION
MARTIAL WAY AND ITS VIRTUES
MASK OF THE KING
MEDITATIONS ON VIOLENCE
MIND/BODY FITNESS
THE MIND INSIDE TAI CHI
THE MIND INSIDE YANG STYLE TAI CHI CHUAN
MUGAI RYU
NATURAL HEALING WITH QIGONG
NORTHERN SHAOLIN SWORD, 2ND ED.
OKINAWA'S COMPLETE KARATE SYSTEM: ISSHIN RYU
POWER BODY
PRINCIPLES OF TRADITIONAL CHINESE MEDICINE
QIGONG FOR HEALTH & MARTIAL ARTS 2ND ED.

QIGONG FOR LIVING
QIGONG FOR TREATING COMMON AILMENTS
QIGONG MASSAGE
QIGONG MEDITATION: EMBRYONIC BREATHING
QIGONG MEDITATION: SMALL CIRCULATION
QIGONG, THE SECRET OF YOUTH: DA MO'S CLASSICS
QUIET TEACHER: A XENON PEARL MARTIAL ARTS THRILLER
RAVEN'S WARRIOR
REDEMPTION
ROOT OF CHINESE QIGONG, 2ND ED.
SCALING FORCE
SENSEI: A CONNOR BURKE MARTIAL ARTS THRILLER
SHIHAN TE: THE BUNKAI OF KATA
SHIN GI TAI: KARATE TRAINING FOR BODY, MIND, AND
    SPIRIT
SIMPLE CHINESE MEDICINE
SIMPLE QIGONG EXERCISES FOR HEALTH, 3RD ED.
SIMPLIFIED TAI CHI CHUAN, 2ND ED.
SIMPLIFIED TAI CHI FOR BEGINNERS
SOLO TRAINING
SOLO TRAINING 2
SUDDEN DAWN: THE EPIC JOURNEY OF BODHIDHARMA
SUNRISE TAI CHI
SUNSET TAI CHI
SURVIVING ARMED ASSAULTS
TAE KWON DO: THE KOREAN MARTIAL ART
TAEKWONDO BLACK BELT POOMSAE
TAEKWONDO: A PATH TO EXCELLENCE
TAEKWONDO: ANCIENT WISDOM FOR THE MODERN
    WARRIOR
TAEKWONDO: DEFENSES AGAINST WEAPONS
TAEKWONDO: SPIRIT AND PRACTICE
TAO OF BIOENERGETICS
TAI CHI BALL QIGONG: FOR HEALTH AND MARTIAL ARTS
TAI CHI BALL WORKOUT FOR BEGINNERS
TAI CHI BOOK
TAI CHI CHIN NA: THE SEIZING ART OF TAI CHI CHUAN,
    2ND ED.
TAI CHI CHUAN CLASSICAL YANG STYLE, 2ND ED.
TAI CHI CHUAN MARTIAL APPLICATIONS
TAI CHI CHUAN MARTIAL POWER, 3RD ED.
TAI CHI CONNECTIONS
TAI CHI DYNAMICS
TAI CHI QIGONG, 3RD ED.
TAI CHI SECRETS OF THE ANCIENT MASTERS
TAI CHI SECRETS OF THE WU & LI STYLES
TAI CHI SECRETS OF THE WU STYLE
TAI CHI SECRETS OF THE YANG STYLE
TAI CHI SWORD: CLASSICAL YANG STYLE, 2ND ED.
TAI CHI SWORD FOR BEGINNERS
TAI CHI WALKING
TAIJIQUAN THEORY OF DR. YANG, JWING-MING
TENGU: THE MOUNTAIN GOBLIN, A CONNOR BURKE MAR-
    TIAL ARTS THRILLER
TIMING IN THE FIGHTING ARTS
TRADITIONAL CHINESE HEALTH SECRETS
TRADITIONAL TAEKWONDO
TRAINING FOR SUDDEN VIOLENCE
WAY OF KATA
WAY OF KENDO AND KENJITSU
WAY OF SANCHIN KATA
WAY TO BLACK BELT
WESTERN HERBS FOR MARTIAL ARTISTS
WILD GOOSE QIGONG
WOMAN'S QIGONG GUIDE
XINGYIQUAN

DVDS FROM YMAA

more products available from . . .

YMAA Publication Center, Inc. 楊氏東方文化出版中心

1-800-669-8892 • info@ymaa.com • www.ymaa.com

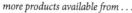

Printed in the USA
CPSIA information can be obtained
at www.ICGtesting.com
JSHW012048140824
68134JS00035B/3324